TEA CLEANSE

Beginner's Guide to Using Tea Detox Diet to Boost
Metabolism

(The Ultimate Guide on the Tea Cleanse)

I0092655

Robert Homer

Published by Sharon Lohan

© Robert Homer

Tea Cleanse: Beginner's Guide to Using Tea Detox Diet to Boost Metabolism (The Ultimate Guide on the Tea Cleanse)

ISBN 978-1-990334-37-5

Legal & Disclaimer

The information contained in this book is not designed to replace or take the place of any form of medicine or professional medical advice. The information in this book has been provided for educational and entertainment purposes only.

Table of contents

Part 1..1

Introduction 2

Chapter 1: Why A Tea Cleanse?...................................3

Chapter 2: What Is A Tea Cleanse? 9

Chapter 3: What Teas To Use For A Cleanse................13

Chapter 4: Benefits Of Tea Cleanse 18

Chapter 5: Now For The Cleanse 21

Chapter 6: Making It Stick...27

Chapter 7: Skin Care Overview...................................32

Know Your Skin 32

Blueprint Of Your Skin...32

Caring For Your Skin 34

Chapter 8: Scrubs...37

Salt Scrubs...38

Salt Scrub Recipes...38

☐   Lavender Lift...38

☐   Casual Citrus 40

Sugar Scrubs..40

Sugar Scrub Recipes 42

Sweet Chocolate..42

Strawberry Sunshine...43

Lemon Honey Treat...44

Jiving Java 45

Conclusion..47

Part 2 48

Introduction 49

Chapter 1: The Caffeine Economy - History and Origins of Tea & Coffee 52

Chapter 2: Tea vs. Coffee - Battle of The Beverages 58

The Digestive System 60

Irritable Bowel Syndrome 60

Heartburn and Acid Reflux 61

Stress and Tension 61

Gamma-aminobutyric acid (GABA) 62

Inhibits Cell Division 64

Lower Cholesterol 64

Destroys Free Radicals 65

Herbal Teas 66

Chapter 3: Tea for Triumphant Weight Loss 69

Slow Metabolism 72

Boosting Metabolism 73

Green Tea 73

Oolong Tea 74

Yerba Maté 74

Goji Tea 74

Chapter 4: Your 14-Day Tea Cleanse Plan 76

Chapter 5: 15 Delicious Recipes for Your Cleanse 83

5 Morning Refresh Recipes 84

Ginger Lemon Honey Tea 84

Tisane Morning Detox Tea 85

Uplifting Morning Green Detox Smoothie 87

Spring Morning Green Tea Detox Smoothie 88

Morning Detox Water 89

5 Daytime Pickup and Detox Recipes..90

Dandelion Tea..90

Milk Thistle Tea 92

Detoxifying Mint Tea..93

Daytime Green Tea Smoothie 95

Cucumber Detox Water..96

5 Evening Colon Cleansing Recipes..97

Peppermint Tea 97

Senna Tea..98

Aloe Vera Juice 99

Psyllium and Bentonite Colon Cleanse Water......................... 100

Good Old Plain Water... 101

Chapter 6: The Tea Cleanse Lifestyle 102

Tea Cleanse Diet Recipes.. 140

Burdock Tea Recipe 141

Garlic Tea Recipe.. 142

Green Fennel Seeds Tea... 143

How To Make Green Tea 144

Fenugreek Tea Recipe 145

Iced Lime Dandelion Tea... 146

Honey-Lemon Ginger Tea Recipe.. 148

Cayenne Pepper Tea With Ginger 149

Matcha Mint Iced Tea.. 150

Lavender Green Tea.. 156

Cranberry Spritzer Green Tea 157

Kiwi and Mango Smoothie Green Tea..................................158

Almond and Blueberry Smoothie Green Tea......................159

Rose Petal Green Tea..160

Tulsi Green Tea..161

Minty Green Tea..162

Peach Mango White Tea..163

Thai Coconut Tea...164

Grapefruit Oolong Tea..165

Vitamin C Tisane...166

Honeycrisp Apple Black Tea...168

After Dinner Digestive Tisane..169

Tummy Taming Tisane...170

Rejuvenating Goji Ginger White Tea....................................171

Nettle Cinnamon White Tea...172

Jack Frost Tisane...173

Rosy Black Tea..174

Autumn Tonic White Tea..175

Lavender Ruby Fruit Lemonade...177

Iced Green Tea with Lavender..178

Peachy Green Tea..179

Refreshing Green Tea with Melon..180

Raspberry-licious Green Tea...180

Green Tulsi Cleansing Tea..181

Green Minty Tea..182

Fruit and vegetable Infused Green Tea................................183

Rosy Green Tea Petals...184

Cranberry Tea Spritzer..185

Green Tea Smoothie 186

Fruity Green Smoothie 187

Conclusion 189

Part 1

Introduction

This book contains proven steps and strategies on healthy weight loss.

Weight loss is a journey and takes dedication. If you have been on every diet in the book and have not experienced the results you are looking for this book has tips that will help you achieve your goals.

The book will explore what a tea cleanse is and how it will help jump start your weight loss. There is a great discussion on the types of teas and what their benefits are. There is a chapter that gives you an easy and good tasting tea cleanse recipe that will help you see results.

More than anything, I want you to be healthy and lose the weight you hope to get rid of. There are several simple things you can do to change your life and turn it around today. Don't delay—read this book and get started toward a new you!

Thanks again for downloading this book, I hope you enjoy it!

Chapter 1: Why A Tea Cleanse?

It is a common fact that our world today is full of toxins. We find them in our processed foods, in our air, in our water, in our clothing—virtually everywhere we go our bodies are bombarded with toxins. The good thing is our bodies were created with their own detoxing organs that process everything we come in contact with. The trouble is the number oftoxins we take into our bodies; the organs get sluggish and we slow down and actually do not feel well. Let's take a brief look at how our organs work to detox the body. This information will be helpful when you actually start your cleanse—you will know and understand what the cleansing ingredients are doing to aid your sluggish organs.

The Body's Detoxing Organs
Kidneys
We know from science that the kidneys detox our blood as well as urine. The toxins are then eliminated from our body through the bladder via urine. It is critical to drink water to keep our kidneys healthy and working properly.

Liver
The liver is one ofthe largest organs in the body (second only to your skin) and has a multitude of functions including breaking down alcohol and other toxins into substances that are not as harmful. It is also

a storehouse for iron, copper and several vitamins such as A, D, E, and K. It also breaks down fat. The liver's main job is to filter blood that comes from the digestive tract. The liver, gall bladder, pancreas, and intestines work together to process food

Lungs

Obviously, the lungs are the organs that give us air. As we inhale the oxygen is passed to the blood. The blood returns carbon dioxide to the lungs where we expel it through exhaling. The hairs in the nose are the first line of defense; they stop large particles from getting into the airway. The way the lungs purify the air is really through little helpers in the respiratory system called cilia–these little hairs stop dust, dirt, and other toxins from settling the lungs by brushing them up and out. Mucus also plays a role in stopping dust, bacteria, and even viruses from entering the respiratory system.

Intestines

Digested food passes through the intestines, nutrients are absorbed, good and bad bacteria find balance, and they produce natural antibiotics that will break down toxins.

Skin

Some folks may not realize the skin is the largest organ of the body. The skin protects the body, but also expels toxins through perspiration.

Lymphatic System

Lymph fluid circulates the body and its white blood cells pick up bacteria and toxins and return them to the lymph nodes. There the toxins are destroyed.

The Human Body & Toxins
Now let's take a look at how toxins affect the human body. Here are some symptoms of toxic overload or having more toxins than your body can efficiently and effectively process. Do any of these sound familiar? Take note: obesity is on the list.

- Achy joints
- Bruising
- Diarrhea
- Digestive problems
- Fatigue
- Headaches
- Irritability
- Obesity
- Poor appetite
- Sensitivity to chemicals
- Sinus problems
- Skin rashes and irritations
- Swelling in the legs

Keep in mind some of these are symptoms of other diseases and problems, so please work with your doctor on this matter.

The way toxins work in our bodies is to keep us off balance. Homeostasis is the ability of the body to maintain balance. Homeostasis can be upset by chemical, biological or physical agents. The human body is very intricate and each organ handles multiple functions. A strong, healthy immune system can typically fight off toxins as they come. But over time, if toxins have damaged the balance, the immune system becomes weak and compromised and we cannot process the toxins like we used to. The toxins begin to build up. The body tries to segregate the toxins so it stores them in the body which appears as cysts, benign tumors, swollen areas, and fat cells. **Take note**: fat cells are storage bins for toxins.

Below is a list of some sources of toxins. How many of them do you use?

- Air fresheners—phenol, cresol, ethanol, xylene
- Dry cleaning spot remover—solvents
- Furniture polish—nitrobenzene, naphthalene, phenols
- Germ killing disinfectants—cresol, phenol, ethanol, formaldehyde
- Heavy metals—mercury and cadmium
- Insecticides—all kinds
- Non-stick pans, ironing board covers, etc.—Teflon; irritant to skin, eyes and respiratory tract
- Oven cleaner—lye aerosols
- Permanent press clothing—resins, formaldehyde
- Personal products like:
☐   Toothpaste—phenol, cresol, ethanol
☐   Cosmetics and mascara- plastic resins, formaldehyde, PVP

- ☐   Talcum powder–some contain asbestos
- ☐   Aerosol hairspray–PVP, formaldehyde
- ☐   Antiperspirants and deodorants–aluminum chloralhydrate, ammonia, formaldehyde
- Prescription Drugs
- Silver polish–petroleum products
- Spray starch–formaldehyde
- Synthetic fibers–nylon, polyester, acrylic- which are all plastics

Since most of us do not live in a bubble, we cannot avoid toxins. The goal is to be free from as many toxins as possible. One area we can start with is our diet; eating"clean", unprocessed foods will go a long way to keeping our organs from bogging down with toxins. Whole foods such as fresh fruit, vegetables, meats and dairy are your better choices and especially if you can buy from local farmers that don't use pesticides or find truly organic products at your local grocery store. The problem with this method is it takes discipline and determination. I believe our toxic bodies make it harder for us to stick to. The following quote is from Dr. Kasi A. Rote who has a medical practice that teaches healthy eating and living. She says,"Give the body what it is asking for. An unhealthy body will crave unhealthy things like chocolate, sugar, white bread, etc... This is a clue as to whether or not your body is healthy. What is it craving? Healthy bodies ask for vegetables, water, protein, etc. Unhealthy bodies crave foods that supply quick, easy energy. This is because a healthy body can derive energy from whole food sources whereas an unhealthy body cannot."

So back to the original question, why a tea cleanse? The purpose of a tea cleanse is to rid one's body of toxins. After reading this chapter it is evident why a tea cleanse may be necessary for some. As far as weight loss is concerned, if toxins are stored in fat cells that hinder weight loss, it goes without saying that ridding the body of these toxins should help with weight loss and bring the homeostasis balance back to the body. It should help maintain a healthy immune system and many other benefits we will discuss in Chapter 5.

We have looked at how the body handles toxins and what some common toxins are, let's look next at what a tea cleanse is all about.

Chapter 2: What Is A Tea Cleanse?

Tea Cleanse—What is it?

A tea cleanse is a safe way to cleanse the body of toxins including your liver, gallbladder, pancreas, intestines, lymphatic system and kidneys in order to have a healthier immune system and a healthier you.

A great detox tea has two steps: a morning refresh tea and an evening colon cleanse tea. The two steps work together to restore balance in your body. The morning tea will reduce bloating; support your metabolism; maintain a healthy immune system, and boost your energy. The evening tea will detox your system; reduce bloating; decrease water retention, and cleanse the digestive system. Finding the right teas for these two processes are critical to success. (There is a review of teas in Chapter 3.)

The initial weight loss comes from ridding your body of toxic waste that has built up in your colon and other vital organs and water weight. The long term results come through changing your diet and adding moderate exercise to your routine. Unfortunately, there is no quick fix to losing weight, but a tea cleanse can be the process that starts you off on a new path.

Tea Cleanse—What it isn't?

A tea cleanse is NOT a way to purge. A tea cleanse is just that, a cleansing before starting a new healthier lifestyle. It is not meant to cleanse and binge and cleanse and binge and so on. In fact, cleanses can be dangerous if you are not doing it with your doctor's permission and not doing it correctly. Constant cleanses can deplete your body of necessary bacteria in the digestive tract that helps with digestion. And, you can become seriously dehydrated. Please, do not use this tea cleanse as a way to purge your overindulgences only to return to indulging. Use it as a way to get back on track, eating healthy, becoming more healthy and feeling and looking better every day.

A tea cleanse is not about starving yourself. It is about being hydrated and changing some bad eating habits for the better. The true purpose of a tea cleanse is to prepare your system for a healthier you. It is to reset the types of foods you will be eating. It is about retraining your taste buds to be satisfied and enjoy more subtle flavors and maybe new flavors and spices. It is not about feeling deprived but about finding clean foods that taste great and satisfy cravings.

Tea cleanses have become a fad and most of them don't live up to what they claim. Be very cautious about what you buy in to; many times you are just giving away your money for something you could have done at home on your own.

Tea Cleanse Do's and Don'ts

In fact, here is a list of some do's and don'ts that may help you understand what a tea cleanse is all about.

DO'S	DON'TS
Do see your physician before starting a tea cleanse	Do not stress out; stress contributes to weight gain and other health issues
Do choose a tea cleanse that is right for you	Don't follow the fad
Do use a tea cleanse as a gateway to a healthier you	Don't indulge; you purpose is cleansing
Do light exercise, like walking	Don't overdo it with heavy, strenuous workouts
Stay hydrated; drink plenty of water	Don't stay up late; go to bed between 9 & 10 p.m.
Eat clean; fresh fruits, veggies, and protein	Don't overeat unless it is green and leafy!
Eat 4-6 lighter meals throughout the day; this will keep cravings at bay	Don't starve yourself

A tea cleansecan be very exciting because you are setting off on a new journey. Take it slow and work through each moment, each day; work toward the success you are looking for. Let's get to Chapter 3 and talk about tea!

http://www.lifehack.org/articles/lifestyle/how-detox-your-body-with-tea.html

http://www.frugallivingnw.com/theultimateguide/

http://www.livescience.com/52524-flavonoids.html

http://www.eatthis.com/5-best-teas-that-boost-your-calorie-burn

http://news.health.com/2013/07/18/planning-a-detox-or-juice-cleanse-5-dos-and-donts/

http://lifehacker.com/what-happens-in-your-body-during-a-cleanse-or-detox-1669540259

http://thechalkboardmag.com/detox-dos-and-donts-10-things-you-should-know-on-a-cleanse

http://news.health.com/2013/07/18/planning-a-detox-or-juice-cleanse-5-dos-and-donts/

Chapter 3: What Teas To Use For A Cleanse

The first thing to know about tea is that green, black, and oolong tea all comes from the same plant; it is the different methods of processing it that give you the different teas. There are also teas that come from different plants such as mint.

When searching for the right tea you need to be sure you get the best ingredients that are fresh, have vitamins and antioxidants, and not filled with toxins of their own. The tea also needs to taste good–whysubject yourself to something that tastes nasty–you won't keep up with the detox and defeat the purpose before you even begin.

Some teahas contraindications, so make sure to do the research so you are not drinking something that is initially good but over the long haul may not be so good. For instance, senna has been shown to stimulate weight loss–exactly what we want; but it has also been shown to cause diarrhea to the point that it depletes your systems of helpful nutrients such as potassium. Others lower blood sugar and shouldn't be taken along with diabetic medication as it can cause low blood sugar. Because tea cleanses are so popular now, a lot of tea has not been fully tested as to the effects they will have on the human body. So, you see, a detoxing tea has many ramifications and it will do you well to make sure the tea you choose will not work against your medications and existing health issues.

This book focuses mostly on green tea because that is the basis for this tea cleanse. But other tea is mentioned so you can become familiar with what is available.

Detox Tea Ingredients and What They Offer

- Green tea:

This fabulous tea has been proven to help burn fat. It contains anti-oxidants. It improves immunity. It has actually been called a super medicine as it has guarded against arthritis, diabetes,and some cancers. It has rehydration properties. Studies have shown it can help prevent neurological diseases such as Alzheimer's.

Green tea contains caffeine, so if you are avoiding caffeine green tea may not be for you. Caffeine has also been shown to be an inhibitor to weight loss. If your goal truly is weight loss then a lifestylechange may need to be made—lose the caffeine. Green tea comes in a decaf version.

Green tea is also an anticoagulant, so may interfere with any blood-thinning prescriptions you may be using.

Green tea works the best when combined with regular exercise. A study at Penn State showed as much as a

27% weight reduction when green tea was combined with exercise. Now that is something to think about!

Here is something else to chew on. A recent study showed drinking 4-5 cups of green tea a day, combined with 25 minutes of exercise lead to losing 2 lbs. more than the group that did not drink tea or exercise.

- Japanese Matcha Tea:

This tea has high levels of antioxidants that fight cancer and destroy free radicals. It is known to lower the bad cholesterol. It helps burn fat. Contain amino acids which help with neurological activities. This tea is similar to green tea but is reported to be ten times stronger.

- Oolong tea:

This tea contains catechins that enhance your body's ability to metabolize fat. It also helps with cholesterol levels. Oolong tea contains many vitamins and minerals that promote health including antioxidants which remove free radicals.

- Mint tea:

This tea helps to curb your cravings. It is actually the aroma of the tea that keeps you from looking for those munchies. Mint also soothes your digestive tract. In addition, it has antifungal properties.

- White tea:

This is the freshest tea and is loaded with antioxidants. White tea also gives fat a one-two punch. It breaks down fat (lipolysis) and blocks the formation of new fat cells (adipogenesis). Sounds wonderful!

- Rooibos tea:

This tea contains a powerful flavonoid called aspalathin. This little feature reduces stress hormones that trigger hunger and fat storage. The Rooibos tea also acts as an appetite suppressant.

- Senna tea:

This tea is made from the leaves of the senna plant which is a herb. The FDA has approved this herb for a laxative. It has also been used in weight loss.

- Dandelion tea:

Dandelion is a natural diuretic helping you lose that excess water weight; but also contains potassium so you don't have to worry about your body being stripped of this important mineral. It also has laxative properties that help you eliminate the toxins that are trapped in your sluggish colon. Loaded with vitamins A and C, plus calcium, this little weed provides a lot of nutrients.

Tea Tips to Follow

Whatever tea you choose, make sure it is a premium tea from a well-known source with a long record of selling tea. The premium teas will give you the most benefits and the freshest taste. Also, buy loose leaf tea as it will have more flavor and stronger health benefits. Store the loose leaves in an air-tight container. The container should not be clear as tea is sensitive to light.

When it comes to premium green teas there are several that always find their way at the top: Bigelow, Stash, Yogi, Numi, Teavana,and Tazo. But just because they are green tea doesn't mean they all taste the same. You may need to do some sampling before you settle in on one that satisfies you. Talk with your friends and see which brand they have chosen. Ask for a sample from them and give it a try.

Do not buy decaffeinated tea. The decaffeinating process typically involves chemicals and rather defeats the purpose of a tea detox program. It is easy to decaffeinate your own tea. Steep it just as you would for normal tea and throw that batch out. Steep again using the same leaves or bags and this 2nd batch will basically be decaffeinated. Water is much purer than any chemicals that would be used to strip out the caffeine.

The steeping of the tea is important as well. If the water is too hot it will damage the tea leaves and reduce the antioxidant effect. If you steep it too long it could also damage the leaves. For tea bags, it is best to steep 1-3 minutes, where loose leaf teas should steep 2-4 minutes.

Finally, sip the tea slowly and enjoy it. So much of life is at a fast pace. The traditional way to enjoy tea is to sip is slowly; take a few minutes for yourself. Tea is not to be gulped.

Chapter 4: Benefits Of Tea Cleanse

Since tea cleanses and detox drinks are rather a fad in today's society there is some controversy whether they actually work or not. My first guess is that they don't work because people don't follow through. Remember, this is about the big picture, about changing some things in our lives so that we become healthier for the long run not just during a 7-day cleanse. If we read the benefits of each and every tea we would be overwhelmed and would hope to drink them all. Clearly, we cannot drink them all, but hopefully, we can settle in on a tea or two that will focus on the areas where we need a boost.

Tea, in general, has many benefits. A recent Harvard study found green tea to have multiple benefits. Green tea is known to reduce the risk of heart disease, help lower cholesterol, lower blood sugar, and fight cancer. It has anti-inflammatory and antioxidant properties. Green tea can also protect the tissues of your eyes, especially the retina. It can help with healthier skin. It can reduce stress. So it seems tea has all the positives that we need to impact our health in a good way. Fill your cup and drink up!

Just so we don't get off track, for the purposes of this book we are looking at weight loss and associated benefits.

Benefits

- Weight loss. The benefit of the tea cleanse is that you are not only ridding your body of toxins, you are ridding your life of poor eating habits and replacing them with healthy ones.

- Rid your body of excess waste. Overindulgences and conditions such as constipation can load your body up with excess waste. You will feel bloated and irritable. A tea cleanse will definitely address this feeling and help things get moving again.

- Natural energy boost. During the tea cleanse you are going to be staying away from toxic foods like sugar and fats. You are going to be adding in fresh healthy fruits and vegetables which will give you an energy boost. Staying well hydrated will also help.

- Stronger immune system. Ridding your body of an overload of toxins frees up your organs to stay on top of moving toxins out of your body as they were meant to do. It will allow your body to absorb nutrients, such as vitamin C, easier giving your immune system a boost.

- Lighter feeling. Ridding your diet of heavy foods that bog down your system will give you a lighter, refreshed feeling.

- Increased health benefits. Research has shown that tea has proven to be helpful in reducing strokes and heart disease; lowering blood pressure; improved mood and weight loss.

- Improved sense of well-being. When you feel good, you have a better outlook on life.

This list of benefits is impressive. Who knew tea was so good for you? The goal of this book is to help you achieve these benefits while you are achieving your goals. So, read on, there is more to come!

Chapter 5: Now For The Cleanse

This is what you have been waiting for: the actual"recipe"for the tea cleanse. As mentioned earlier, this tea cleanse will be a two step process and last one week (7 days). Here are a few ground rules before we get to the cleanse itself.

- You must drink water to stay hydrated. Tea has a diuretic effect and you could become dehydrated if you do not drink plenty of water throughout the day.

- During the detox, avoid drinking soda, juices, and alcohol. These beverages add extra sugar and other toxins to your body, basically undoing what you are trying to accomplish.

Green Tea Cleanse

Step 1: The Morning Tea

We are going to use a green tea. In Chapter 3 I mentioned the brands of organic green tea that are considered premium and the best to use. These include Bigelow, Stash, Yogi, Numi, Teavana, and Tazo. These teas are reasonable in price and most readers should be able to find one of these green teas. Most of these green teas also come with a flavor, such as mint. Choose a flavor you enjoy. They also sell sample packages so you can try several flavors and settle in on one or two.

There is also the Japanese Matcha Tea, which is also available from several premium brands. Matcha is quite expensive so I opted not to go with this one. If your budget allows, go for it. This tea is thought to be heavier in antioxidants and other benefits.

Steep the tea for 3 minutes. Drink 8-10 ounces (no sweeteners or other additives). I suggest you make this sort of a morning ritual. Set aside an extra 5 minutes where you can sit quietly, sip your tea, and maybe plan your day or read something inspiring. This will set your day on the right path and begin to remove the toxin of stress from your life. At the end of drinking your tea, do a few deep breaths. This will fill your lungs and exhale out the toxins. Inhale as you raise your arms up; hold for a few seconds; exhale as you bring your arms down. Do this 4-5 times. Add in some stretches as well.

This will seem very new to you and maybe even silly as you breathe and stretch. But you will begin to see results. Trust me.

Step 2: The Evening Tea

Again we are going to use an inexpensive, yet pure premium tea that is easy to find. The detox teas have all the wonderful properties and benefits as green tea, plus some added extras. You will note the teas listed below all include dandelion. Some of its properties were mentioned in Chapter 3. One other feature of note is that dandelion raises the enzymes that help with the detox process. The ingredients in the detox tea will begin to work on your digestive tract and begin removing the toxins that you take in from your food.

Of the premium brands we discussed earlier, only a few offer a true detox tea. There are other detox teas brands on the market such as Fit Tea, Bootea, Lyfe Tea and Tiny Tea. Actually,there are probably hundreds of different teas on the market. But one precaution—not all teas are organic or made the same. Some detox products are scams. So if you choose to go with a detox program make sure you know what you are getting into.

- Bigelow—Bigelow does not offer a detox tea at this time

- Stash

ü   Pure Detox Tea: Tulsi, dandelion root, mulberry leaf, sarsaparilla, safflower, lemon oil, wintergreen oil

- Yogi

ü   DeTox Tea: Indian sarsaparilla root, organic cinnamon bark, organic ginger root, organic licorice root, organic burdock root, organic dandelion root, cardamom seed, organic clove bud, organic black pepper, juniper berry extract, organic long pepper berry, Phellodendron bark, organic rhubarb root, Chinese skullcap root, Coptis root, forsythia fruit, gardenia fruit, Japanese honeysuckle flower, winter melon seed ü   Roasted Dandelion Spice Tea: Organic roasted dandelion root, organic dandelion root, organic cinnamon bark, organic cocoa shells, organic cardamom seed, organic ginger root, organic clove bud, organic black pepper.

- Numi–Numi does not offer a detox tea at this time

- Teavana–Teavana does not offer a detox tea at this time

- Tazo–Tazo does not offer a detox tea at this time.

Make this your bedtime ritual. Steep the tea for 3 minutes. Drink 8-10 ounces (no sweeteners or other additives). Drink slowly and go over the events of the day, letting them go and letting go of the stress that comes with them, When finished with your tea do some simple slow stretches, reach for your toes 4-5 times; do some arm circles about 10 times; do some torso twists 4-5 time and end with deep breathing 4-5 times. This should prepare you for a great night's sleep.

Follow this tea cleanse ritual for 7 days and 7 days only.

Step 3: The Ground Rules

By now you realize the tea cleanse is not just about drinking tea for 7 days. It is about making changes in all areas of your life that need to be rid of toxins. Weight loss is very complex. All sorts of things affect weight loss: food, emotions, relationships, self-esteem, and so much more. My goal is to help you reach your goal. Since I don't know each and every reader and your individual situations I am giving some guidance so you can take the extra step and make it work for you.

- Get the"okay"from your doctor before proceeding with the tea cleanse.

- Weigh yourself at the beginning. Weigh yourself at the end. Do not weigh yourself in between. Somehow seeing that number on the scale is very defeating and sabotaging. Wait for it...

- During the tea cleanse you need to rid yourself of sugars, trans fats, saturated fats, and processed foods as much as possible. This means clean eating: fresh fruits, vegetables, and proteins. This does not mean starving. The average woman should eat about 1,500 calories a day to lose one pound per week. The average man should eat about 2,000 calories a day to lose. I know you want to lose weight fast; but, slower is better. During the tea cleanse eat enough calories to sustain your body. Chances are 1,500-2,000 calories are going to be a lot less than you have been eating. You may see a significant drop the first week.

- Do not overeat. The goal is to lose weight and the simple math is we cannot overeat. The math formula is calories in–calories out = gain/loss. So, if you eat 2,000 calories in a day but only burn 1,500 calories through your daily routine and exercise, you have a net gain of 500 calories which will lead to weight gain. You always want the calories burned side of the equation to be greater than the calories in, that way you will see a net loss.

- Follow the tea cleanse for only 7 days. You do not want to deplete your system of essential nutrients and bacteria. You do not want to be dehydrated. The tea cleanse is meant to be a jump starter to a healthier you, not a long term program. The long-term program comes after the 7-day cleanse, where hopefully you will continuing making healthy choices and seeing healthy results.

- Do light exercises. This will help circulate the lymphatic fluid through your body helping it to drain and taking the toxins with it.

Chapter 6: Making It Stick

If you are like many in the US, you are constantly on a yo-yo diet. You go down; you go up and so on. It gets very frustrating and makes you want to give up. The good news is with just a few easy changes and some determination you can see positive results that will last. And, if you have done any research on losing weight or have tried the many fad diets you must accept the truth–there is no overnight fix. Chances are it took you several years to pack on the pounds. It will take several months of hard dedication to see results. But don't give up–you can do it!

Clean Eating

In Chapter 1 we talked about toxins and how they come from a variety of places. When it comes to weight loss your biggest toxins are going to come from food. Here are the two biggest culprits: sugar and gluten (flour). The principal behind clean eating is that you eat whole foods. Cutting out sugar and flour is not an easy task, but the rewards will be great. You will be a much healthier person and a much smaller person.

What are whole foods? These foods are not processed: fresh fruits, vegetables, and meats/proteins. When you eat whole foods you can eat a large quantity because it is low in calories and high in nutrients that feed your body. Avoiding toxins are the key that means foods such as prepackaged meals; lunch meats; breaded and fried anything; cakes, cookies, and brownies; pasta and the like. There are many clean eating cookbooks available with recipes for things such as flourless cake or grilled shish kabobs with veggies and shrimp. The possibilities are endless.

My recommendation to you is to start eliminating some of those processed foods that your body craves and replace it with something"clean". For example, trade apple pie for a baked apple with cinnamon and raisins. Trade pasta lasagna for eggplant lasagna where thin slices of eggplant are the noodles. This is delicious. Each week cut out something and trade it for something fresh. You will be surprised by the results.

Stay Hydrated

Our bodies really are amazing organisms. They have all the power to keep you healthy and balanced. You have taken the leap to do a tea cleanse and start over with a clean slate. You are cutting out the processed foods that bog down your system with toxins. You also need to stay hydrated and this means with water. Caffeinated drinks, alcohol, sodas, and juices should no longer be on your daily beverage list. Water and tea will be your mainstay and on weekends or for special occasions add in a special beverage.

Moderate Activity

The words workout or exercise probably drive most of us crazy. We don't have time, we don't know what to do, we can't do it or basically we don't want to do it. The truth is our bodies were made to move. If we take a trip back into history we see where mankind at one time was hunters/gatherers/farmers meaning they did physical work basically for the purpose of eating. So imagine working out 8 hours every day just to get your one meal for that day. In those days most people with of healthy weight, strong and muscular. Fast forward to today and we have instant gratification. We can drive to the ice cream store at night for the hot fudge sundae and the most work we did for it was put on our shoes. See the difference? Our bodies are made to move.

Now, that being said studies have shown that three 10-minute workouts are better and more effective than one 30-minute workout. That is exciting! We don't have to carve out great chunks of time to work out. What's more, moving or exercising doesn't have to mean 30 minutes on the treadmill. How about vacuuming or mopping your floors–maybe that takes 10 minutes. How about walking the dog–there areanother 10 minutes. How about doing a few exercises while you watch your favorite television program–there arethe final 10 minutes. So, with just a little creative thinking you can get some extra moves in during your regular day. Don't make it harder than it is.

Miscellaneous Helpful Tips

There are several tips that are worth reviewing because the goal of this book is to help you be successful and I want you to have all the tools necessary to meet your goal of losing weight.

- Do not set yourself up for failure. One example, clean your cupboards of processed foods; chips, sweets, bread, and such all have to go. If you leave them in your house you will eat them and you will feel bad. You will get discouraged and quit. It is a vicious cycle—almost as bad as coming off a drug; it could be worse for some people.

- Do not let your spouse or partner sabotage you. It is sad to say, but if your partner is not on the same path as you concerning getting healthy and losing weight, they will try to sabotage you. It may be subconscious, but it will happen. Be prepared. Have your response ready. Don't give in. Some of this comes from an insecurity or jealousy that once you get thin and healthy you will leave them. Some of it comes from control, they want to be in control of what you do and who you are. So, when they invite you out to a nice dinner be prepared to suggest a place that serves mostly clean food or at least to a place where you can get something good to eat such as a nice salad (hold off on the dressings) and a piece of lean meat. You've got this, so don't give in.

- Find a friend who you can be accountable to. If we try to do things alone we sometimes struggle or fail because we feel all alone. We feel like no one knows what it is like to be in this spot in life. Find a friend that you can confide in, talk with weekly or daily if need be, has a listening ear and will encourage you. In a way,it is like having a sponsor. The time you head to McDonald's for a Big Mac, call your friend and let them talk you out of it.

- Journal: This may be a bit overused, but journaling really can help. You can record your feelings on any given day. What you have struggled with. Definitely, write down your victories. This will tell your story and help you as you live it.

- Reward yourself when you meet a big goal (not with food, but maybe some new shoes or something you have wanted for a long time)

- Don't give up! During this process,there will be ups and downs. When you fall down, get up and start again. Don't let your body win by giving in; let it win by overcoming food and becoming healthy.

We have covered a lot of territory in this book. Some of it may be overwhelming. Some of it may be exciting. I want you to know that these techniques work because I have done it.

Chapter 7: Skin Care Overview

Everyone wants to have beautiful skin. We want to look our best, especially as we age and we begin to see wrinkles appear. With the health and fitness craze, we are concerned about our cardio health, our bones, and other organs. Did you know that your skin is the largest organ of your body? What!? Yes, your skin is an organ that works to protect your body. Let's look at some facts about the skin that I think might surprise you.

Know Your Skin

Your skin is ever changing and regenerates itself every 27 days.

The skin is a covering that protects us from germs. The white blood cells in your skin are created to attack invaders such as bacteria. Your skin tells your body to activate the immune system.

Your skin also regulates your body temperature. The blood vessels work together to contract or expand depending on the temp.

The nerve endings in our skin allow us to feel heat, cold, pain, pressure and texture. The skin signals the brain to let it know what we should be feeling. It all happens in just milliseconds!

Blueprint Of Your Skin

Your skin has three layers: the epidermis, the dermis, and the hypodermis. Each has its valuable function.

The top layer is the **epidermis**. The central part of the epidermis is keratinocytes that produce keratin. The melanocytes produce melanin which is the pigment that colors your skin.

The next layer is the **dermis**. It has connective tissue and is home to hair follicles and sweat glands. Sweating is good for you; it keeps you cooler and carries out impurities and toxins. The nerve endings are also in the dermis. The nerve endings are what allows you to feel textures, temperatures, and pain. There are also glands in your skin that make oil. The oil produced by these glands is a natural protection for your skin making it waterproof. The oil is present in the epidermis. Sometimes your body will produce too much oil which could cause pimples or blemishes.il which could cause pimples or blemishes.

The **hypodermis** is what you might call a fat layer. However, it has essential duties to fulfill. It attaches the skin to the body, muscles, and bones, through the use of connective tissues. This layer is also important in helping to regulate your body temperature. Blood vessels and nerve endings that start in the dermis travel through the hypodermis to other essential parts of the body, like your brain and your heart. Finally, the fat is also a protector, insulating your muscles and bones from bumps and simple falls.

So now you see the importance of the skin. Not only does it protect and purify our bodies but it interacts with other organs to keep everything functioning well.

Caring For Your Skin

Toxins and pollutants run rampant in everyday life. These things affect our health, yes the health of our skin. Toxins make our skin age faster. Our skin is constantly battling on our behalf to keep germs, bacteria, viruses, and toxins out of our bodies. The more we subject our skin to these poisons, the more our skin ages. our skin to these poisons, the more our skin ages.

Consider the cosmetic and beauty products you use. Have you ever read the labels? Do you know what you are putting on your skin that is being absorbed by your body? From shampoo to deodorant, to lotions, to foundations, to lipstick, to soap—it all has harmful chemicals in it. Unless you are using 100% organic products, there is a high chance you are using something that is doing more harm than good. Removing harmful chemicals from our lives is the central premise of"clean living."You want to not only put clean foods into your body; you want to use clean ingredients on your body and in the environment around you. This lifestyle is not easy—yet. Clean, organic products are not readily available in many areas of our country. The movement is growing, and I have seen chain grocery stores adding in many more organic and clean selections for food and other things.

If you adopt this way of life, you will be on the cutting edge of a fast-growing movement. This movement is fighting against genetically modified organisms (GMO) in our foods. Clean living and utilizing organic products is a huge step toward healthier living."clean living."You want to not only put clean foods into your body; you want to use clean ingredients on your body and in the environment around you. This lifestyle is not easy–yet. Clean, organic products are not readily available in many areas of our country. The movement is growing, and I have seen chain grocery stores adding in many more organic and clean selections for food and other things. If you adopt this way of life, you will be on the cutting edge of a fast-growing movement. This movement is fighting against genetically modified organisms (GMO) in our foods. Clean living and utilizing organic products is a huge step toward healthier living.

So, how can we take care of this large organ that protects us and works to keep us healthy? There are several common sense things we can do to help our skin.

● **Hydration**: The skin, along with the rest of your body, needs water to hydrate and get rid of impurities.
● **Sleep**: We have all heard of beauty sleep, and it is true! While we sleep, our skin works to repair itself. Collagen production is at its highest while we are sleeping.

- **Nutrition**: Yes, your skin benefits from eating right.
- **Cleansing**: Our skin is bombarded throughout the day with a variety of pollutants and impurities. Be gentle to your skin and keep it clean on a regular basis.
- **Sunscreen**: Protect yourself from harmful sun rays. Use sunscreen if you have to be outside during the hottest times of the day. Use SPF15 as a minimum.
- **Don't smoke**: The pollutants and impurities from smoke will cause your skin to age faster.

We want to emphasize using organic products in all our recipes. The main reason is your skin is a protector and will fight against anything that may be harmful. There is no need to use possibly toxic ingredients that may have chemicals or pesticides in it. Organic products are better for you because your skin will absorb these moisturizing products. Organic products will not harm the environment either. When you bathe, the residues from your lotions go down the drain. Organic products will not harm the ground water like products with a variety of chemicals. Choose to live"clean."n. Organic products will not harm the ground water like products with a variety of chemicals. Choose to live"clean."

Chapter 8: Scrubs

There are some fantastic recipes for salt scrubs and sugar scrubs. Both types of scrubs are exfoliants. The purpose of an exfoliant is to remove dead skin cells. Aside from removing dead skin cells, there are several other benefits which are very inviting.

- Improved circulation: the scrubbing motion and pressure will encourage your body fluids to increase and even correct the flow.
- Improved reduction in cellulite: the scrubbing motion on cellulite prone areas can reduce the appearance of the cellulite. Scrubs utilizing a coffee base are quite helpful in this area.
- Anti-aging: removing the dead skin cells is going to give you a glow and reduce the appearance of fine lines.
- Absorbs moisturizer: Using a scrub on a regular basis and following it up with a moisturizing body lotion is the best treatment. Your body will be able to absorb the moisturizer better having the dead skin cells removed. You will have smoother, healthy skin.
- Relaxation: in today's hurry and scurry world, anytime for relaxation is coveted. A body scrub is relaxing because you are taking time out for yourself and treating yourself to a treatment that is healthy and beneficial to you.

Safety Note: If you use these scrubs in the bath or shower, be aware that the oils can make the surface of your tub or shower very slick. Put a hand towel or dish towel in the bottom of your tub or shower to stand on. It will help you prevent a fall.

Most of us love going to the spa, but our budgets will not let us go as often as we like. You can recreate the spa right in your home. Since you will be making the products, you know the ingredients will be the best you can find. Add some soft music, a few candles and create the spa-like atmosphere right in your bathroom.

Salt Scrubs

First of all, salt scrubs have deeper exfoliant powers just by the nature of more abrasive granules. Secondly, sea salt gives added benefits of minerals such as magnesium and potassium. Salt scrubs are great for reducing inflammation, relieving symptoms of arthritis and can reduce tension.

Some folks will find that salt can be a bit irritating to their skin, so it is best only to use a salt scrub about once a week. Using a finer salt granule may also help with any irritation. Here are a few salt scrub recipes that your skin will love!

Salt Scrub Recipes

☐ Lavender Lift

- 1 cup sea salt (Himalayan pink sea salt has 84 trace minerals that will be great for your skin)
- ½cup nourishing oil such as grape seed, almond, or avocado
- 5-10 drops of lavender essential oil
- Dried lavender petals and leaves (this is optional but does add some color and more fragrance to your scrub)

Mix and store in a glass jar. Pretty up the jar with a lovely lavender ribbon. This recipe is very versatile. You can add any essential oil and change it up. Peppermint is a great one to use on your feet. Put in a clean, dry jar.

Lavender essential oil has many benefits, but one of the most well known is its calming effects. If you have tension or stress in your life, lavender can lift your spirits and mood. It gives you a sense of peace and relaxation. Lavender is also an excellent acne fighter and healer. First it works to stop bacterial growth on the skin, second, it helps to regulate the glands that secrete oils, so there is no overproduction, and finally, it soothes and heals the red, irritated skin.

☐ **Fancy Face**

This salt scrub is so easy with just two ingredients. Mix equal portions of sea salt and extra virgin olive oil. Put in a clean, dry jar. Apply to your face (or whole body) but be careful not to get too close to the eyes. Wash off alternating between cold and warm water.

☐ Casual Citrus

- ½cup sea salt
- ½cup nourishing oil
- ½teaspoon lemon zest
- ½teaspoon orange zest

Mix these ingredients together and store in a clean, dry jar.

Citrus is excellent for use on your skin. It has moisturizing properties and also is a great toner. Citrus is good for you, inside and out.

☐ Mocha Madness

If you like the smell of coffee and chocolate, then this salt scrub may just become your favorite. Check out the recipe.

- ¾cup sea salt
- ½cup nourishing oil
- ¼cup unsweetened cocoa or¼cup freeze dried coffee
- One teaspoon vanilla extract
- Two tablespoons of honey

The honey has healing properties and also will give added moisture as part of the end results of this scrub. Store the scrub in a clean, dry jar.

Sugar Scrubs

A sugar scrub will feel wonderful and leave your skin looking fresh and clean but does not have the added minerals that salt offers. The granules of sugar are smoother and won't provide the stronger exfoliant powers, but will still do a great job. It is safe to use a sugar scrub 2-3 times a week.

The most important thing to remember about sugar scrubs is they have a short shelf life, especially if you have added any fresh fruit. You can store your scrubs in the refrigerator which may give you a little longer shelf life. Here are a few sugar scrubs that will be very yummy for your skin!

Sugar Scrub Recipes

Sweet Chocolate

- ½cup organic coconut oil
- ½cup safflower oil
- 1½cups organic brown sugar
- 1 Tablespoon organic raw cocoa powder
- 1 Tablespoon maple syrup or honey

Mix the coconut oil and safflower oil together for a few minutes. You are looking for a creamy texture. Add in the brown sugar a small portion at a time. Add in the cocoa and honey or syrup. Mix thoroughly. Put in a clean, dry jar and store in the refrigerator.

Cocoa has antioxidant compounds and is great for your skin. It can repair damaged cells and protect cells in advance. Cocoa also includes a variety of vitamins including A, B, D, and E.

Strawberry Sunshine

- ½cup organic coconut oil
- ½cup grapeseed oil
- 1½cups refined organic sugar
- A handful of freeze dried strawberries (scrub will last longer) or fresh strawberries chopped
- 5-10 drops sweet orange essential oil

Mix the coconut oil and grapeseed oil thoroughly. Slowly add in sugar. Mix to get a creamy texture. Add in strawberries and essential oil. Mix thoroughly. Put in a clean, dry jar and store in the refrigerator.

Strawberries have exfoliating properties and contain alpha-hydroxy acid that helps take care to dead skin cells. They also have salicylic acid which helps reduce dark spots and tightens pores reducing acne breakouts.

Lemon Honey Treat

- 1 cup organic cane sugar
- ¼ cup olive oil
- 2 Tablespoons raw honey
- 2 Tablespoons dried lemon zest
- 10 drops lemon essential oil

Mix sugar, oil, and honey thoroughly. Add lemon zest and lemon oil. Mix. Store in a clean, dry jar.

Honey and lemon are great for your skin. They contain anti-inflammatory and antibacterial properties which fight against blemishes. They also are an excellent skin toner. Honey will help keep your face moisturized and supple.toner. Honey will help keep your face moisturized and supple.

Jiving Java

- 6 Tablespoons finely ground organic coffee
- 4 Tablespoons organic coconut oil
- 2 Tablespoon turbinado sugar
- One teaspoon organic vanilla extract

Melt the coconut oil; add in other ingredients. Stir until thoroughly mixed; store in a sealed jar. This scrub will last up to 2 months.

There are plenty of benefits in a coffee scrub. Coffee contains anti-inflammatory properties. A good scrub will help reduce eye puffiness (don't get too close); improve your circulation, and give you beautiful smooth skin. The caffeine in coffee will help tighten the skin. It is also loaded with antioxidants to help fight wrinkles and fine lines. Caffeine is also a stimulant. So here's a chance to wake up your body and mind - have a cup of coffee before your morning shower. Then, give yourself a great coffee scrub. You will be ready to start your day refreshed and renewed!

There you have some great salt and sugar scrubs with which to start. Make sure to go easy on your skin and don't use these scrubs too often. Try once a week for salt scrubs and 2-3 times on the sugar scrubs max. Make sure to use fresh, organic ingredients and take note of which recipes work the best with your skin.

These scrubs also make lovely gifts. Store them in beautiful jars and add a fancy ribbon and a little doodad. Voila! You have a great homemade gift and an excellent way to express your creative side!

Conclusion

A tea cleanse may be the perfect jump start to making healthier choices in eating, exercising and living. While there are many benefits it is not to be continued over the long term. The recipe given in this article spans several days and then you stop. The weight loss will come through the change in diet and the addition of exercise. On the other hand, knowing what we know about green tea and all its benefits it is fine to drink green tea (decaf version) moderately and gain all that you can from it. Best wishes to a healthier you!

Thank you for downloading this book, I hope it was able to help! The next step is to try to remove daily toxins that come from processed foods and eat more whole foods. In addition, add some easy to moderate exercise such as walking. Before you know it, you will see results.

Part 2

Introduction

This book has actionable steps and strategies on how to lose weight, improve your health, increase energy, remove toxins, and speed up your metabolism by going on a tea cleanse diet.

We live in a polluted world; the air we breathe, the water we drink, the foods we eat and everything we come into contact with has traces of various pollutants. Unfortunately, many of these substances somehow end up into our bodies. While our bodies have an inbuilt mechanism designed to get rid of all the wastes, the truth is that with the ever increasing level of exposure to various toxins or pollutants, our body's natural detox mechanism cannot match the amount of toxins that we feed into these systems.

And like any other system, if the balance between input and output is disrupted, the only thing you can expect from that is chaos. Think about it; since our bodies cannot cleanse themselves naturally, either because we are exposing them to toxins that the body cannot process for elimination or because what we are exposing our bodies to is too much for it to handle, there is likely to be various problems.

These problems relate to excessive toxins accumulation within our bodies. Some of the problems that come with too much toxicity within our bodies include chronic fatigue, rapid weight gain coupled with the accumulation of fat around the belly, deteriorated health, difficulty losing weight and lots of other problems. Over time, these problems can result to various health complications like diabetes, cancer, chronic inflammation, metabolic syndrome and many others. As such, if you are to combat or avoid the health complications that come with increased toxicity within the body, the only way to do that is through 'helping' the body's natural detox process since this will enable you to get rid of the toxins that have build up within your body. You can only live a healthy life when you don't have an excessive toxin buildup within your body.

So what is it you can do to 'help' the body to detox? Well, while there are many things you can do to boost the body's natural detox, diet is undoubtedly the one surefire way through which you can get this done. In particular, taking something that you are already used to taking will definitely make the process of adopting a detox diet very easy for you. That's where tea comes in. Do you know that you can use various kinds of teas to supercharge your body's detox process and in so doing derive all the benefits that come with being free from toxins? Well, you can. And this book will show you exactly how tea can help you detox, the different kinds of teas that you can use to detox, the properties that are in different teas that enable them to boost your body's natural detox and much, much more. When you read this book, you will realize that there is more to tea than the fancy name and its refreshing aroma.

Thanks again for downloading this book, I hope you enjoy it!

Chapter 1: The Caffeine Economy - History and Origins of Tea & Coffee

Fascinating Beginnings

If you're a superhero fan by any chance, you'll understand the value of a good origin story.

The very fact that you're interested in reading this book probably means you partake in at least some tea or coffee drinking. Maybe you're enjoying a cup right now?!

But, it's likely that you haven't ever explored the origins of what you're drinking which is why this chapter exists. You're about to learn all about where tea and coffee really come from!

History of Coffee

Legends and mythology are always fun and fascinating. It's true for the legend that tells how coffee was first discovered. It's said that an Arabian goat herder by the name of Kaldi, noticed that after his goats nibbled on a dark green-leafed plant with bright red berries, they were dancing about with new energy. After witnessing the event on several occasions, the goat herder decided it must be the berries on this particular plant.

His curiosity got the best of him and he decided to try them himself. It was at that moment he learned of their power to stimulate. The secret, as the story goes, was shared with the local monks at the monastery who used the stimulant to help keep them awake during long prayer sessions.

While such legends stay around for centuries, recent botanical evidence tells a slightly different story. New evidence shows that the coffee bean's history found its origins in the plateaus of central Ethiopia around the 6*th* century. From Ethiopia the beans were brought to Yemen and it was there that coffee plants were first cultivated.

As the love of the beverage took hold, the first coffee houses sprung up in Cairo and Mecca. How interesting that coffee became a passion and a social event early on.

The early variations of coffee used the whole raw bean. It wasn't until the sixteenth century that the bean was roasted, which brought in a whole new flavor of coffee.

The plants were closely guarded by the Arabs who saw the advantage of having the corner on the market. However, by the 1600s, seeds had been smuggled out of the country and the Dutch were able to start coffee plantations in Sri Lanka and then Java.

From the Dutch, the idea of maintaining vast coffee plantations in the tropics spread to France, Spain, then finally to the Colonies in the 1700s.

The colonists, at the outset were tea drinkers – having brought the custom over from Britain. However, after the tax on tea because a divisive issue between the colonies and Great Britain (remember the infamous Tea Party), tea quickly went out of fashion, and coffee took its place.

As the westward expansion took place in America, coffee went right along with it. A pot of coffee over the campfire became part of the environment of the wagon trains, and later of the cowboys herding cattle out on the range.

Anyone remember taking the "coffee break" at work? For an entire era in post-WWII America, in nearly every workplace, a few minutes a day was designated as a coffee break. Coffee was definitely ingrained into the culture by that point.

The most recent phase of the coffee evolution in the US has been coffee shops serving espresso, and all manner of coffee specialty drinks. Such places (think Starbucks) have created a trend not only for social occasions, but for the individual who wants to set up the laptop, connect to the Wi-Fi, and get a little work done in a relaxing atmosphere. The growth and popularity of coffee shops – both chain stores like Starbucks, and little mom and pop setups – has been nothing less than phenomenal.

But we've gone down this coffee road as far as we're going to for this book. Now we'll change focus and find out the history on tea.

History of Tea

One can hardly even think of the word tea without the vision of Brits enjoying their daily afternoon tea. Tea time has been ingrained in their culture for several generations. But tea certainly didn't originate in England.

This time, for this origination legend we travel to China rather than Arabia. The legend tells us that the Chinese emperor Shen Nung was sitting outside while his servant was boiling water. Leaves from the nearby tree happened to blow into the water. Because Shen Nung was a famous herbalist, his curiosity was aroused, and he decided to taste the concoction. When he found it to be tasty and enjoyable, the new beverage of tea was born.

The tree happened to be a Camellia sinensis which is a species of evergreen shrub whose leaves and leaf buds are, to this day, used to produce tea.

All legends aside, the reality is that mentions of different types of teas are found in Chinese writings as early as 350 BC. Either way, the point is that tea originated in China and it happened a very long time ago.

It was in the twelfth century that traveling Buddhist monks brought tea to Japan. In that country, tea drinking was elevated to a solemn ceremony thus it became deeply entrenched into the Japanese culture.

When tea traveled to Europe in the 1600s, it was first touted as a medical drink only. But when a Portuguese princess, Catherine of Bragaza, married Charles II of Britain in 1662, she brought tea and served it to friends at court. Once royalty added their stamp of approval, the custom grew and spread. Soon there were tea gardens all across London.

In the 19th century, Anna, the Duchess of Bedford, came up with the idea of offering tea and snacks to afternoon guests. Hence the origination of afternoon teatime in Britain. For the upper class it became the bridge between the midday meal and supper, which might not be served until 8PM. And of course, it was served with great ceremony with splendid tea wares.

As mentioned in the history of coffee, tea went out of favor in American during the Revolutionary War. From then on tea took a back seat to coffee as the American beverage of choice for many decades.

The popularity of tea picked up when the idea of iced tea was introduced – especially in the south. (To a tea connoisseur, iced tea isn't really tea at all, but that's another subject.) For a tea lover in America, it's difficult to find an eating establishment where you can get a decent cup of tea. That now is changing.

Starbucks has recently purchased Teavana, and tea cafes similar to Starbucks are springing up in many metropolitan areas. In addition, tea shops that carry a vast array of exotic teas are also catering to tea lovers.

In correlation with the rise in tea drinking has come the discovery of some of the amazing health benefits of teas. The most interesting of which – and the subject of this book – is healthy and natural weight loss.

Now that you've learned the history of these two popular beverages, we're going to turn the discussion of the benefits (or lack thereof) of both. Information that is crucial for optimum health.

Chapter 2: Tea vs. Coffee - Battle of The Beverages

Preface to The Battle

For many decades, to most Americans, tea was tea. If you wanted a cup of tea you bought a package of tea bags and it was usually *black pekoe* tea. The selection ended there. Then a company from Boulder, CO emerged on the scene offering *herbal teas*. Starting in 1969, this company, Celestial Seasonings, changed the way most people thought about a cup of hot tea. Now there were flavors which before were unheard of in a tea. Lemon, raspberry, chamomile, mango, apple, peach, and the list goes on and on.

One line of their teas was dubbed *wellness teas*. This proved to be a new idea and a new concept. Consumers began drinking green tea to stave off cold symptoms, peppermint tea to calm an upset stomach, and chamomile tea to help get a good night's sleep, and so forth. Grocers and specialty shops couldn't keep them on the shelves. (Especially in flu season.)

While Celestial Seasonings was a pioneer in this field, many other companies have since picked up the baton and latched onto this successful venture.

But even with all this talk about wellness teas, is it true that tea is healthy and good for your overall health?

And is it better for you than coffee? In short: is tea healthy and coffee unhealthy? To get the answers to those questions, we have to get into the proven research. We'll start with coffee.

Coffee: An Overview

Coffee is without a doubt America's favorite beverage. Statistics tell us that about 180 million people start their day with a caffeine jolt from a cup of coffee. While many people can drink coffee for years and never have any issues, there are others who suffer from several potential negative effects. The worst of these is when it becomes so addictive that the person cannot bear to go a day without it.

For the individual who drinks an occasional cup of coffee, and if that coffee is organic and of a high quality, it's true that there can be benefits. (And it's especially important that it be organic since coffee is one of the most pesticide-intensive crops on the market.)

Studies have shown that coffee improves alertness and over the long term it may reduce the risk of developing Parkinson's disease, gallstones, kidney stones. It can also work as a preventative against liver cirrhosis for those who are heavy drinkers. High quality coffee has also shown to provide antioxidants which help fight free radicals in the body. Again, this has been proven only with the consumption of high-quality coffee.

The problems arise because the majority of coffee drinkers are not having an *occasional cup*, and what is consumed is far from what could be considered as high quality. Especially the type that comes out of the typical vending machine, or the coffee maker in the company office.

Many negative health issues are contributed to coffee consumption, actually too many to list in this book. But let's look a few of the more major issues.

Pros and Cons of Coffee

The Digestive System

The human gut is able to digest food due to the gastric acids that are secreted within the stomach. One of these is called *hydrochloric acid*. Coffee introduced to an empty stomach stimulates hydrochloric acid secretion – which is usually what happens when the coffee drinker awakens each morning – they down a quick cup of coffee first thing.

If the stomach is forced to secrete excess gastric juice because of the coffee, it may become deficit when it comes time to digest the protein eaten at lunch and dinner. Protein entering into the small intestines that is not completely digested can cause a wide variety of serious health problems. Many diseases can be traced back to the gut, which means it's crucial to keep it as healthy as possible.

Irritable Bowel Syndrome

Coffee also has been shown to irritate the lining of the small intestine. Such irritation can lead to abdominal spasms, cramps and elimination problems – this causes alternate issues with constipation and diarrhea. This condition is known as *irritable bowel syndrome* (IBS) and the number of people diagnosed with this malady is on the rise.

Heartburn and Acid Reflux

Once a person has finished eating a meal, a small bundle of muscles at the lower end of the esophagus (known as the *lower esophageal sphincter*) is designed to tightly close. This prevents the contents of the stomach from moving back up into the esophagus and burning the lining with hydrochloric acid.

Coffee becomes problematic because it relaxes this set of muscles. (As does some colas and high-caffeine energy drinks.) Distressful heartburn and acid reflux can be the result. Even decaf can cause heartburn in some people due to this relaxation of the lower esophageal sphincter muscles.

Stress and Tension

For many coffee drinkers, the reasoning behind their habit is the *jolt* needed to keep them going - to ward off the mid-morning drowsies, or for an extra kick while working on a project late into the night.

It's true that coffee promotes the release of stress hormones such as cortisol, epinephrine and norepinephrine. These chemicals are especially designed to be released in dangerous situations so that the body's heart rate, blood pressure and tension levels will shoot up. It's the *fight or flight* response.

While most coffee drinkers say they want a shot of energy, for many the pattern has moved past that and into a revved-up chemical imbalance that causes a jumpy, jittery feeling. It's this sensation of being wound up which makes it difficult to relax. Yes, the coffee stimulant will help you through the late-night project, but the concern should be the long-term effects on overall health. Increasing the chemicals for the fight-or-flight response hinders normal digestion. If a person is in a genuinely frightening situation – say an accident – the body is smart enough to cause digestion to cease during the *shock* time. For coffee drinkers this occurs every day.

Gamma-aminobutyric acid (GABA)

Another problem area with coffee is GABA metabolism. GABA stands for Gamma-aminobutyric acid. This is the neurotransmitter that assists in regulating stress levels. It also has a calming effect on the gastrointestinal tract. Coffee interferes with the metabolism of GABA.

It's interesting that a person's mood and digestion are so closely interconnected. And yet, a heavy consumption of coffee negatively affects both of these areas.

As I mentioned, health issues linked to coffee make up a long list, but from what has been included here, hopefully, you can get a clearer understanding. Now let's get a more detailed understanding about tea.

Tea: An Overview

We can't really begin a discussion about tea without understanding that there are many different types of teas:

- _White Tea
- _Green Tea
- _Oolong Tea
- _Black Tea
- _Herbal Tea
- _Rooibos Tea
- _Blooming Tea

The good news is that health benefits can be found in each of these types of tea. While some teas contain caffeine, it's a much lesser amount than coffee. Plus the fact that its effects last longer and without the downer often experienced with coffee. This is especially true with green and white tea, since they are brewed for shorter times and at cooler temperatures.

Additionally, *L-theanine*, an amino acid which is found only in tea, tends to relax the body without reducing alertness. This is opposite to the jitteriness caused by caffeine in coffee.

Already we can see a major difference between the two beverages, and an important benefit in tea. Let's look at a few other benefits.

Pros and Cons of Tea

Inhibits Cell Division

The flavonoids found in many teas have been found to lower the risk of certain cancers by inhibiting free radicals and some carcinogens. Tea also promotes programmed *cell death*, or *apoptosis*. As it inhibits the rate of cell division, that in turn, decreases the growth of abnormal cells. (Cancer is the growth of abnormal cells.)

Lower Cholesterol

Extensive studies have shown green tea to be helpful in lowering cholesterol levels. This includes both serum cholesterol and LDL. The studies showed that five or more cups of green tea a day led to the biggest drops on the cholesterol levels.

Anti-inflammatory

It's becoming increasingly well known that inflammation can be connected to a wide range of ailments such as arthritis, metabolic syndrome, and depression. The active compounds found in tea help lower levels of inflammation. This can be related to heart problems since cardiovascular disease can be directly linked to inflammation. Thus we can assume that drinking tea is good for heart health in addition to overall health of the entire body.

Allergies

Quercetin is a flavonol that is found in tea which eases histamine response. Histamine is responsible for the body's natural allergic reaction to certain allergens such as pollens. (Which is why antihistamines are purchased over-the-counter for relief of allergies and cold symptoms.) Tea becomes the natural, healthy alternative to drugs.

Destroys Free Radicals

Oxidation of free radicals in the body is a process that increases risk for diseases such as heart disease, cancer, Parkinson's disease and Alzheimer's. Tea just happens to have the ingredients needed to fight free radicals.

Tea is high in *oxygen radical absorbance capacity* (ORAC), which tells us that it helps destroy free radicals in the body. Our bodies are designed to fight free radicals on their own, but they're not always totally effective, plus the fact that we live in a toxic world that continually adds to the free radical levels. Tea can be part of the answer in the daily fight to rid our bodies of harmful free radicals.

Herbal Teas

Herbal teas differ from other tea in that they are derived from plant leaves, seeds, roots or bark, which are then extracted in hot water. Drinking a well-steeped cup of herbal tea, we get the full impact of the plant's benefits in an easily digestible drink. Below is listed a few different types of herbal tea:

• Peppermint tea

• Ginger tea

• Chamomile tea

• Rooibos tea

• Lemon balm tea

• Rosehip tea

Some aid in digestion, others have a calming effect, still others work as detox and cleansers. So many wonderful herbal teas to choose from. You can start with a couple and try them out to see which ones are best suited for your tastes and your needs.

How to Switch From Tea to Coffee

You've read enough to convince you that you really could (or should) make the switch from coffee over to tea. But how? Especially with such a strong dependency on coffee, not only in the body's system but also the psychological addiction.

First of all, don't think of it as giving up something. View it as launching into a new adventure. Go slow. No need to get in a hurry. Begin slowly with a substitution here and there. Say you start your morning with three cups of coffee each day. Begin to trade one out for a cup of tea, the next week trade out two cups. And in the third week allow all three to be cups of soothing, relaxing tea. At the same time, introduce a cup of hot tea as your after-dinner beverage.

Coffee lovers who have made the switch say that black teas suited them better at the beginning, simply because they have a stronger taste. Some of the *breakfast teas* are great for a morning pick-me-up. This would include English breakfast tea. They're a blend of the stronger black teas and they may use Assam tea leaves as well. (This refers to tea from the Assam district of India). This produces a tea that is pungent, malty tasting, and full-bodied. Because it's darker than most teas, it appears more like coffee.

Earl Grey is another possible choice for making the switch. It's a unique-tasting tea that is scented with the oil of bergamot. It's mild-flavored, yet the taste is very distinctive.

How you start is not really that important; what matters is that you're serious, and that you're ready to kick the coffee habit. This isn't to say that coffee is inherently bad. It is not. But an addictive cycle that controls your life is not a good thing no matter how you look at it.

Now that you've become familiar with the basic information about tea and coffee, and all the many health benefits of tea, let's go past that to the fact that these health benefits can include weight loss. We'll talk about that in the next chapter.

Chapter 3: Tea for Triumphant Weight Loss

Why Coffee Contributes to Weight Gain

Before going into the relationship between tea and weight loss, we need to return to the subject of coffee again momentarily. You will remember it was stated that coffee produces chemicals in the body that replicate the *fight or flight* behaviour and this includes the chemical *cortisol.* Cortisol increases blood sugar levels, and this in turn is converted into fat.

Studies show that when cortisol levels are raised for a prolonged amount of time, the body must relocate fat deposits from other parts to the abdomen. Many of us have heard the term *beer belly.* Sorry to break the bad news, but there is also such a thing as a *coffee belly.*

Add to this the fact that the majority of coffee drinkers load their beverage with milk and sugar which increases the calories. And don't forget the sweet treats that go *so good* with a cup of java. When it comes to the subject of weight gain, few people take their coffee into consideration, but it can be a huge factor.

The Relationship Between Weight Loss and Health

It's a sad fact that many dieters are more concerned with how many pounds are being lost than the overall health of their body. The truth is that good health has a lot to do with whether the pounds go or stay.

The point here is that different varieties of tea have different health and healing properties. This alone is a great reason to consider tea as part of your weight loss plan.

Health Benefits of Green Tea

For this discussion, we're going to focus on green tea. We've already discussed the fact that green tea contains a large amount of beneficial substances. One of these is caffeine – which is much less than in a cup of coffee. The caffeine in green tea aids in fat burning and aids in exercise performance.

The best part about green tea, however, is its wide variety of antioxidants – green tea is loaded with potent antioxidants called catechins. The most beneficial of these is EGCG (Epigallocatechin gallate), a substance that boosts metabolism.

Another great thing about green tea is that you can purchase what is known as *green tea extract*. This is a food supplement that can increase your daily intake for more powerful weight loss effects.

The active compounds in green tea aid in the process of breaking down fat cells and moving them into the bloodstream. It actually boosts the effects of some of the fat-burning hormones in the body.

Yet another function of EGCG is that it slows down an enzyme that breaks down the hormone *norepinephrine*. To interpret, that simply means that levels of norepinephrine increase. More norepinephrine creates a stronger signal being sent to the fat cell and more fat gets broken down. The synergistic effect of both caffeine and EGCG found in green tea enhances this process even further. When the fat cells break down more fat, which is then released into the bloodstream, it becomes available to other cells, such as muscle cells.

In the body we have different types of fat. One is the subcutaneous fat – this is fat that lodges right under the skin. But we also have what is known as visceral fat – this is the belly fat that builds up around the organs. Of the two, it's the latter that is more harmful. It can cause inflammation and insulin resistance which are linked to serious diseases such as type 2 diabetes and heart disease.

The studies done on weight loss effects of green tea emphasize the fact that it's the harmful visceral fat that is lost, which is great news. Now we're back to pointing out the importance of good health as well as weight loss. This type of weight loss can mean a reduced risk of killer diseases, which can lead to a longer and healthier life.

Metabolism: How It Contributes to Weight Loss and Gain

Slow Metabolism

A huge factor to consider in weight loss is a person's metabolism. Metabolism refers to all of the biochemical and hormonal reactions in the body necessary to keep organs and cells working.

Basal metabolic rate (BMR) tracks the minimum energy it takes your body to burn the maximum calories. Your BMR will account for 40-70% of the energy your body needs daily to maintain this rate. The percentage depends on factors such as weight, age, and amount of activity in your lifestyle. When someone says they have slow metabolism, what they are really saying is that they have a low BMR. For the sake of our discussion, we'll stick with *metabolism* since it's the term that's most familiar.

What causes metabolism to slow down? There are several reasons, but at the top of the list would be inactivity. Muscle cells burn more calories than fat cells. The muscle mass on an inactive person tends to shrink and metabolism goes down.

Highly restrictive diets can also slow metabolism over time. As a survival mechanism, the body lowers its basal metabolic rate when food is restricted. (Most dieters believe just the opposite.)

Age is yet another factor. As the cells in the body age, they slow the pace at which they use energy.

Boosting Metabolism

On the converse side, let's look at what causes metabolism to speed up. Exercise is the main booster of metabolism, so when the body exerts energy, extra calories are burned. Remember we said that muscles cells require a lot of energy. This means the BMR goes up when the muscles are put into action.

Next on the list, after exercise, would be change in the diet. Because fiber absorbs fat, it's good to eat a diet rich in fiber to boost metabolism.

And in keeping with the theme of this book, let's touch on the different types of tea that boost metabolism.

Metabolism Boosting Tea Types

Green Tea

Green tea contains catechins, an antioxidant that enhances the release of fat from fat cells. This, in turn, speeds the liver's capacity for turning fat into energy. (Keep in mind there's a big difference between actual green tea, and the bottled stuff with added sugar.)

Oolong Tea

Like green tea, oolong is also packed with catechins, which boost weight loss efforts by improving the body's ability to metabolise fat.

Yerba Maté

Yerba Maté (yer-bah mah-tay) comes from the leaves of the South American rainforest holly tree. It is said to be as strong as coffee, and yet as beneficial health-wise as tea. Of the most common stimulants (such as coffee, tea, and cocoa) yerba maté is the most balanced because it delivers both energy and nutrition.

This tea offers powerful thermogenic effects, which helps turn up your body's calorie-burning mechanism.

Goji Tea

Dried goji berries are easy to find in your local health food store, but there is also a goji tea available. The plant from which goji berries are harvested, is a traditional Asian medicinal therapy, but it also offers a slimming effect.

Preparing a cup of tea is so simple. All you need is a cup of hot water and a teabag. Or loose tea and a small tea strainer. Simple, quick, easy. Very little fuss or bother, and right in front of you there you have a delicious and enjoyable way to boost your own metabolic rate and help you lose weight.

In the next chapter we'll add yet another benefit of tea in your life and that is for a detox, or cleanse. Check this out.

Chapter 4: Your 14-Day Tea Cleanse Plan

Detoxification: What Exactly It Does for Your Body

A cleanse for your body is also known as *detox* (detoxification). We live in an environment saturated with toxins. They're in the air, the water, our foods, and even in chemicals in our homes. Entering into a periodical cleanse time is not only great for weight loss, but is essential for optimum health.

Reasons to seriously consider a detox plan are many and varied. Here are just a few.

• ____Detoxing removes harmful toxins from the body

• ____The cause of many diseases such as cancer, heart disease and strokes, can be traced to environmental toxins. While our bodies have a built-in detox function, that function is often overloaded and needs help. Detoxing assists the body to do that and as a result helps prevent disease.

• ____Regular detoxing strengthens the body's immune system and thereby fights off infections such as those that bring on colds and the flu.

• ____Bodies that are loaded with toxins are not functioning at peak performance. Problems such as joint pain, stomach distress, insomnia, fatigue and so on, are rampant. Getting rid of toxins through a regular detox program and can eliminate many of these health maladies.

•____Detoxing improves energy levels, both physically and emotionally. Sleep patterns are improved and less sleep is needed. The person with added energy is more eager to get involved in an exercise program.

•____Another problem with toxins is that they affect the body's ability to burn fat. Detoxing help the body to get rid of toxins stored in fat cells. This increases metabolism and enhances weight loss.

Now that the reasons for a cleanse is clearer, you might be wondering what does tea have to do with a detox plan? Let's take a look.

Tea Cleanse Diet and Psychology

It's important to have the right mental attitude for a two-week cleanse. The idea is not a *diet,* but a rest. There will be foods to avoid, but only for two weeks. You want to give all the organs of your body a rest – a chance to renew and refresh. Detox tea will play an important role, but no successful cleanse can depend on a drink alone.

Check your calendar and select two weeks where there are no special social events so you can remain consistent.

Avoid:

- ***Alcohol***
- ***Cigarettes***
- _Milk products

- _Sugar, honey, maple syrup, artificial sweeteners

- ***Coffee***
- _Grains: wheat (bread, biscuits, cakes, pasta), rye, barley, oats, spelt and rice

- _Dried fruit

Enjoy:

- _Any and all fresh fruit

- _Any and all fresh vegetables

- _Fresh or canned (in water) fish

- _Lean red meat, chicken – two servings each week

- _Dried or canned legumes such as kidney beans, chickpeas, lentils

- _Eggs (organic is best)

- _Olive oil (preferably extra virgin),

- _Coconut oil (unprocessed)

- _Raw unsalted almonds, walnuts, macadamias and cashews

- _Raw unsalted sesame, pumpkin and sunflower seeds

- _Green tea, white tea, weak black tea (decaffeinated)

•_From one to three liters of water per day

During the first few days of detox you may experience a reaction which can include headaches or loose stools. These symptoms are perfectly normal (although not all that common) and should subside in 24 to 48 hours if you do experience them. They are merely a sign of the body adjusting to a new routine.

Once your diet is clean, detoxifying teas will enhance your natural organ function.

You'll find a number of detox teas on the market, some with complete daily plans for how to use the teas in your detox plan. Some of these include:

•Detox Dandelion

•Lemon & Ginger

•Yogi DeTox

•Lemon Jasmine Green Tea

Daily Tea Schedule for Best Results

As you start your 14-day plan you will begin each day with a tea that refreshes the body and replaces lost vitamins and electrolytes from the evening colon cleanse tea. (More about that later.) Your *refresh* tea should contain a blend of ingredients that have high levels of anti-oxidants and vitamins.

Having your colon cleanse tea is how you will close out each day of your 14-day tea cleanse. The mixture will contain ingredients such as:

•<u>Senna</u>

•Dried orange peel
•Dandelion plant
•Nettle leaf
•Lemon grass
•Liquorice root

Begin the day with your refresh tea, end each day with your colon cleanse tea. Throughout the day, enjoy multiple cups of hot tea. Try rotating the teas mentioned to enhance the detoxing process. During your cleanse, eat small meals using the foods from the above list.

What to Expect From Your Tea Cleanse

Due to the radical change in eating habits; due to the colon cleanse and the detox effect, it is possible to lose a pound a day during your 14-day detox plan (*14 pounds in 14 days*), much of which is lost is from previous water retention and excess buildup in the colon.

This rate of weight loss is not only possible, but highly probable. Again, a word of caution – it's best not to enter into a cleanse with a *diet mentality.* Such a mindset can add a measure of anxiety. The true goal of the cleanse is a rest for the entire body, and that includes your emotions. So sit back and relax and allow your body to do what it's designed to do and that's building toward optimum health.

In the next chapter, you'll discover 15 delicious tea recipes which you can enjoy every day of your cleanse.

Wrapping Up Your Tea Cleanse
During your 14-day cleanse your digestive system has been resting, healing, and getting rid of damaging toxins. Avoid thinking of the end of the cleanse as a calorie holiday. Go with foods that are easy to digest and avoid heavy starches, sugars, and fried foods. It's best to choose foods carefully for at least three days following the last day of your cleanse.

Just before moving on, check this out. This same section is copied in at the end of the book also but if you're feeling excited and looking forward to starting your tea cleanse, it may be worthwhile for you to consider this now.

We live in a time when people's schedules are busier than ever, and free time is often at a minimum. Maybe you know what I'm talking about?

That's why it's important to make things as easy and simple as possible for yourself through the use of certain tools. Think about it - you use online email services to send messages all across the world, no need to physically write out a letter, package it and send it via some expensive and sometimes-unreliable courier service. Just one example of how modern technology makes your life easier and more efficient. Below, I've listed some useful tools you may want to consider investing in to make your tea cleanse (and active lifestyle) smoother and more efficient also:

FitBit Activity Tracker: Essential for calorie tracking and optimising your workouts. *NutriBullet 12-Piece High Speed Blender:* The best tool for making those delicious smoothies and fresh juice drinks!

TRX Suspension Trainer: The ultimate portable workout tool, use it to burn calories and work out anywhere, any time. *Hamilton Beach Coffee Brewer:* You may be transitioning away from coffee to tea, but that doesn't mean toucan't enjoy a cup as part of your cleanse!

Fit-Tea 14 Day Herbal Tea Pack: If you're on a tight schedule and need a quick, easy pre-made detox tea, Fit-Tea is still the best choice.

Chapter 5: 15 Delicious Recipes for Your Cleanse

In this chapter, you'll discover 15 recipes which are delicious and functional. There are 5 recipes to use for your morning refresh, 5 for a daytime pickup and metabolism boost and 5 for evening colon cleansing - fulfilling the schedule outlined in chapter 4.

Along with the tea recipes which will be the cornerstone of your cleanse, there's also some detoxifying water and smoothie recipes included which will work as an effective substitute to tea if you fancy a change, or don't have time to brew tea during the morning rush!

Stick to tea as much as possible though, as the techniques discussed in this book are designed mainly to work with tea :)

5 Morning Refresh Recipes

Ginger Lemon Honey Tea

Ingredients:

- __4 cups of water
- __1-2 piece of ginger peeled and sliced
- __Fresh-squeezed juice of 1 lemon
- __1 tbsp of honey

Boil the water.

Add ginger to hot water; simmer for 5 to 10 minutes.

Remove from heat and add lemon juice and honey.

Mix well

This will be your go-to morning refresh tea recipe. Have a cup of ginger tea each morning to regulate metabolism, stimulate digestion, and reduce cortisol production. For the best results enjoy at least 2 cups of your ginger tea each day.

Tisane Morning Detox Tea

Ingredients

- ___6-inch piece of fresh ginger
- ___1 teaspoon of turmeric
- ___2 cinnamon sticks
- ___1/2 teaspoon of cayenne
- ___spoonful of raw honey
- ___squeeze of lemon

Peel the ginger and slice thinly on the diagonal.

Add ginger slices to a saucepan with 6 cups of water and bring to a boil.

Turn to a low heat and simmer for 10 minutes.

Add the cinnamon sticks, cayenne and turmeric, then simmer for another 10 minutes.

Strain into a mug.

Stir in the spoonful of honey and squeeze of lemon.

This recipe is similar to the one before, but with a bit more spice! Don't overdo the cayenne or turmeric otherwise it may be a bit too spicy.

Again, enjoy two cups per day - one first thing in the morning and another mixed in with your daytime metabolism boosters.

Uplifting Morning Green Detox Smoothie

Ingredients

- ___1 Cup of Water
- ___1/2 Cup of Chipped Cucumber
- ___1 Cup of Strawberries (frozen if possible)
- ___1 Banana - optional (frozen if possible)
- ___1 Cored Apple
- ___2 Tightly Packed Cups of Spinach
- ___Juice of 1/2 Lemon
- ___Ice (if not using frozen fruit, or if you want an extra chilled smoothie)

Throw everything into your blender and let it run until smooth!

This green smoothie will give you a massive morning energy boost and kickstart your metabolism for the day ahead.

It's also high in vitamin A, vitamin C, fiber, iron, manganese, magnesium and potassium.

Spring Morning Green Tea Detox Smoothie

Ingredients

- ___1 Cup of Green Tea - Chilled
- ___1 Cup of Loosely Packed Cilantro
- ___1 Cup of Loosely Packed Baby Kale
- ___1 Cup of Cucumber
- ___1 Cup of Pineapple
- ___Juice of 1 Lemon
- ___1 Tablespoon of Fresh Ginger - Grated
- ___1/2 Avocado

Same as the last recipe - throw everything straight into your blender and run until smooth. Nice and easy!

This is a great detoxifying smoothie to start your day - a mix of savoury and sweet flavors which will also give you a slight boost of caffeine from the green tea.

A perfect source of energy and cleansing for a busy morning.

Morning Detox Water

Ingredients

- __12 Ounces of Warm Water
- __Juice of 1/2 Lemon
- __2 Tablespoons of Apple Cider Vinegar
- __Dash of Cayenne Pepper

Add the ingredients to a glass, stir well and enjoy!

Avoid using hot water, as this will kill the essential properties of the ingredients. Stick to warm water only, and you may want to add up to a teaspoon of organic honey at first until you get used to the tartness of this drink.

Wait 10-15 minutes after finishing this drink before eating anything, so that your body gets the chance to properly absurd the nutrients.

5 Daytime Pickup and Detox Recipes

Dandelion Tea

Ingredients

- __1 Cup of Boiling Water
- __1 Teaspoon of Fresh Dandelion Leaves
- __Dash of Honey

Pour the boiling water over the dandelion leaves, let steep for 3 minutes, stir then let step for another minutes. Add a dash of honey to sweeten and enjoy!

Once you pick the dandelion leaves, wash then thoroughly and refrigerate inside a plastic bag with holes punched in it for better air circulation.

Use them up as soon as possible since they are quite perishable.

Dandelion tea is a delicious mid-day treat with potent liver detoxifying properties. It also contains lots of antioxidants like vitamins A, C and D as well as significant amounts of zinc, iron, magnesium and potassium.

So long as you can find some fresh dandelion leaves, it's easy to make and can be rotated in with other daytime tea recipes as you like.

Milk Thistle Tea

Ingredients

- ___One Tablespoon of Milk Thistle Seeds

- ___3 Cups of Boiling Water

Crush one tablespoon of milk thistle seeds in a mortar and add 3 cups of boiling water. Steep for about 20 minutes and strain

A super straight-forward recipe which is great 30 minutes before a daytime meal. It contains an ingredient called sylmarin, which is a combination of three flavonoids that are potent antioxidants responsible for protecting and repairing liver cells.

Detoxifying Mint Tea

Ingredients

- ___4 Teaspoons of Coriander Seeds

- ___4 Teaspoons of Fennel Seeds

- ___1 1/2 Teaspoons of Whole Cumin Seeds

- ___2 Teaspoons of Black Peppercorns

- ___3 Ginger Slices - 1/4 inch Thick

- ___16 Fresh Mint Leaves

- ___3 Thin Slices of Lemon

Combine the coriander seeds, fennel seeds, cumin deeds and black peppercorns in a jar, stir well and set aside.

Bring two cups of water to a simmer. While the water is heating, pound the ginger with the mint to break it up a bit. Use a mortar and pestle, or use a wooden spoon or cocktail muddler.

When the water is hot, stir in 1 tablespoon of the dry mixture and the ginger-mint mixture. Simmer for 3-5 minutes, remove from heat, cover, and allow to steep for another 3 minutes or so. Place the lemon slices in a strainer, and strain the tea through the lemon into a pot or container.

This is another tea with strong detoxifying properties, which you can drink throughout the day and features somewhat peppery taste thanks to the black peppercorns and ginger.

Daytime Green Tea Smoothie

Ingredients:

Make a cup of strong green tea and store in fridge until thoroughly chilled. Once cold, pour it into a blender and then add:

- ___1/8 Teaspoon of Cayenne Pepper

- ___2 to 3 Tablespoons of Freshly Squeezed Juice of 1 Lemon

- ___2 Teaspoons of Agave Nectar (or honey)

- ___1 Small Pear, Skin On, Cut Into Pieces

- ___2 Tablespoons of Fat-Free Plain Yogurt

- ___6-8 Ice Cubes

Blend until smooth. Enjoy as a mid-afternoon picker-upper.

Cucumber Detox Water

Ingredients

- __3/4 Glass of Water
- __3 Ice Cubes
- __2 Slices of Lemon
- __1 Slice of Grapefruit
- __2 Small Slices of Lime
- __3 Slices of Cucumber
- __6 Mint Leaves

First add the water and ice to a glass, then throw in the rest of the ingredients.

Stir and let it sit for 5 minutes, and keep the ingredients in the glass as you drink.

This detox water drink is another simple recipe with minimal prep time. The cucumber provides a refreshing taste while other ingredients give a major energy and metabolism boost.lo

5 Evening Colon Cleansing Recipes

Peppermint Tea

Ingredients

• __1/4 Cup of Mint Leaves

• __Boiling Water

Pour boiling water over the leaves, steep for 10 minutes and strain out the leaves before serving.

This is one of the most simple recipes you'll find, however it is also very effective.

Drink in the evening, shortly before bed for colon cleansing. Peppermint tea is also packed with antioxidants, and helps sooth the stomach, ease sore throats and relieve heartburn if you happen to be experiencing any of those symptoms!

You can add a dash of honey or maple syrup as a sweetener if you like.

Senna Tea

Ingredients:

- ___One Teaspoon of Dried Senna or Three Tablespoons of Fresh Senna Leaves

- __8 Ounces of Boiling Water

Add the dried senna or senna leaves (whichever you're using) to 8 ounces of boiling water, steep for 5-10 minutes, strain and drink!

Senna tea has been used as a medicine in Arabic and European countries since way back in 800 BCE, mainly as a laxative.

It's this laxative property that will help cleanse your colon and remove unwanted buildup of toxins and other junk.

Aloe Vera Juice

Ingredients

• __Juice of 1 Lemon

• __Fresh Aloe Vera Gel

Add the juice of 1 lemon to fresh aloe vera gel and put the mixture in a blender to make a few ounces of smooth juice. Refrigerate for 2-3 hours before drinking and consume shortly before bed.

Aloe vera is a potent detoxifier and acts as a laxative, which is why it's regarded as an effective colon cleanser. Not only will it improve the health of your colon; it will also treat other health issues like headaches, skin infections, diarrhoea, gastric pain and constipation.

Not a tea recipe, but still super effective.

Psyllium and Bentonite Colon Cleanse Water

Ingredients

- ___1 Rounded Teaspoon of Psyllium Husk

- ___1 Teaspoon of Bentonite Clay Powder or 1 Tablespoon of Liquid Bentonite Clay

- ___8 Ounces of Water

Place the psyllium and bentonite in an empty glass, add water and stir briskly. Drink quickly before it thickens, and follow it up with another 8 ounce glass of plain water to help circulation.

If you choose to try this recipe, drink it 2 hours apart from any supplements or medication and at least 1 hour before heading to bed.

Good Old Plain Water

Ingredients

- __Plenty of Water!

Ok, this isn't really a recipe but after going through a full 14-day detox, your going to want to keep your colon clean and let it do its work naturally.

If you go beyond 14 days of evening colon cleansing, your body may start to rely on it to help waste elimination which isn't ideal. Therefore, drinking plenty of clean water every day will help keep your colon clean long-term and avoid buildup of harmful toxins.

Aim for at least 8-10 glasses of water per day and your colon will stay healthy and efficient for a long time after your cleanse!

Chapter 6: The Tea Cleanse Lifestyle

Further Optimising Your Tea Cleanse
The best way to optimise your tea cleanse is to find the tea flavors that you prefer. At the outset you'll want to try several of the ones mentioned so far in this book. As you experiment you'll find the ones that are the most pleasant to you, both in flavor, and in their effects on your mood and your body.

Do your research to learn more about the origins and the benefits of each type and blend of tea. Find a tea shop near you that carries a wide variety of teas, and then discover and experiment. Shop owners usually know which teas are best for a healthy cleanse.

Fitting Tea into Your Life
If you are the coffee connoisseur who never gave tea a second thought, this could be a whole new approach for you. Or perhaps you thought of tea only as a tall glass of iced tea with your meal at your favorite restaurant.

Hopefully, after reading through this book, your ideas about tea are changing. You now understand more about not only the health benefits of tea, but also how tea can easily fit into your weight loss program. And which tea to choose to accomplish that goal.

The best way to fit tea into your life is to simply jump in and try it. Begin trading out a cup of coffee each day for a cup of tea, and build up from there. What a great day it will be when your coffee jitters (caffeine jitters) are a thing of the past.

Can You Drink Too Much Tea?
Too much of anything is probably not good. Reason and common sense needs to come in to play. Because there are so many different kinds and types of tea, it would be rather difficult to consume too much.

But again, use common sense in your selection of tea and in the amount you consume and any dangers will be eliminated. It would be far more probable that one could drink too much coffee than to drink too much tea.

Scheduling Regular Tea Cleanses
Using tea as a way to cleanse your body for better health, for added energy, and for weight loss, is a great addition to anyone's health plan. Once you've experience a 14-day cleanse plan, and once you learn how much better you feel, you'll want to schedule such events on your calendar. You certainly don't want to make this a once-in-a-lifetime event.

A good plan might be to have two such major cleanses each year, and have a shorter weekend cleanse once a month, or once a quarter. Choose whichever one fits into your lifestyle and your schedule.

The key is to begin to think of your tea detox times as a *way of life* for you. Once you begin to experience greater energy levels, more restful sleep patterns, better health (fewer colds, allergies, and bouts with the flu), plus pounds being shed, you'll be sold on your tea cleanse.

Getting Started

What Exactly Are Toxins?

In simple terms, a toxin is anything that has the ability to cause damage to the body; it (toxin) could come from the food we eat (e.g. legumes and wheat), from the air we breathe if it is polluted, the water we drink when it is polluted, mold, clothing, and from literally anywhere. As I stated in the introduction, when you are exposed to toxins, some of these toxins find their way into the body through different channels. And since the body has its own mechanism of removing toxins, it starts eliminating the toxins to stop/prevent them from causing harm to the cells, organs and organ systems. So what exactly is detoxification?

What Is Detoxification?

Detoxification simply means cleaning of the blood, a natural process that our body participates in to transform, neutralize and get rid of unwanted materials; our bodies eliminate toxins through the kidneys, intestines, skin, lymph and lungs. Unfortunately, when the detox process is compromised, the impurities end up not being properly filtered and this affects every cell in our body.

In this context, I will talk of detoxification to mean improving and optimizing the general function of our bodies by supporting our natural detoxification and elimination system while reducing the amount of toxins that gets into our system.

To get us started in this learning journey, let's first understand how toxins affect us just to spur your motivation to get started:

How Toxins Affect Our Health

As I already stated, toxins could be anything that interrupts your normal psychology and impacts the functioning of your body in a negative way. The rate at which we expose ourselves to chemicals keeps growing at an exponential rate and has become a part of our lives today. The different toxins that we are exposed to can be divided into two: endotoxins and exotoxins.

Endotoxins are toxic substances bound to the wall of our bacterial cells and are usually released when the bacterium ruptures. Lactic acid, uric acid and ammonia form part of the endotoxins. They are general wastes from our cells' normal activities. When these toxins build up, they end up causing diseases. A good example is gout, caused by uric acid.

Exotoxins on the other hand are toxins secreted by a bacterium. They cause major damage by destroying the cells or disrupting normal cellular metabolism in the host that carries them. Exotoxins are human-made toxins that we expose ourselves knowingly or unknowingly. They are found in skin-care products, cleaning products, air fresheners, house paints, curtains, prescription drugs, food packaging, processed foods, emission from cars and industries, kid's toys and even the tap water we drink.

The result of exposure to these toxins manifests itself daily as different health problems. Some symptoms that may show that you have high levels of toxins in your body include allergies, digestive problems, diarrhea, constipation, bowel irregularities, depression, low energy, skin issues and headache. Some toxins can kill the friendly bacteria in our guts, interfere with DNA synthesis, block oxygen from binding to red blood cells, block the enzymes the body needs for normal function or block the absorption of vitamins and minerals.

Normally, our detox mechanism is capable of getting rid of the toxins that find their way into the body. For instance, once the liver breaks down toxins, they have to be excreted by the kidney, the skin or via the bowels. Unfortunately, and due to our heightened exposure to toxicity all around us, the rate at which we accumulate toxins is a lot higher than the rate at which the organs responsible for cleansing our bodies can get rid of these toxins. When that happens, this results to what is referred to as bioaccumulation. For instance, a case like constipation can place an excessive burden on the bowels while overworked kidneys begin to fail as toxins accumulate over years. Worse still, the accumulated toxins are the ones that cause irritation and damage. This is known as toxic overload and has been proven to result to all manner of health complications some of which will be discussed below:

Some chronic diseases linked to toxins buildup include:

1. Obesity

This is undoubtedly one of the common effects of increased toxicity within the body. Many toxins linked to obesity are endocrine disrupters. Fat cells act much like endocrine organs usually release hormones related to your appetite and metabolism (fats are responsible for secreting leptin and ghrelin hormones i.e. the satiating and hunger hormones respectively). This makes them a target too for endocrine disrupting toxins.

In addition, toxins accumulation within your body can cause the body to store more fat cells in order to bind these toxins and keep them away from the major vital organs. For you to understand this (and other effects of toxins) better, perhaps it is important that I mention that toxins are of two broad types; water-soluble toxins and fat-soluble toxins. The water-soluble toxins are easily removed through the skin (through the sweat glands as sweat) and the kidneys (through urination). The kidney, liver, skin, colon and lungs are the major detox organs in our bodies. Unfortunately, the fat-soluble toxins (often referred to as xenobiotic compounds) are not that easy to remove. So how are these eliminated?

Well, when the detox process is working optimally, it all starts with the bile being secreted from the gallbladder. The liver does not only synthesize and secret bile, but it also acts as a filter for bacteria and toxins in the blood and chemically neutralizes them then converts them into substance that the kidney can easily eliminate. The purpose of bile is to sort of 'dissolve' (by converting it into a water soluble form as shown in the next paragraph) the fats thus making it easy to absorb them through the intestinal villi into your lymphatic tissue. This region has a high concentration of white blood cells, which usually responds to the toxicity.

Supposing we could divide the detox process into two phases: the first one by the liver and the other by the gastrointestinal tract and the kidneys, then this is how the natural detoxing process takes place. The liver helps in detoxing in two ways. First, cytochrome pathway enzymes turn the fat-soluble toxins into intermediate toxins, which happen to be more hazardous than the fat-soluble versions. Conjugation pathway enzymes then turn the fat intermediate toxins to a water-soluble toxin ready to be excreted and marking the end of the first phase.

The second phase is quite complex. The gastrointestinal tract, which allows toxins to enter for excretion is pH sensitive. The toxins must therefore be in the right PH before being accepted for further processing. As the toxins move in the gastrointestinal tract, they interact with billions of bacteria living in the there. If the ratio of the healthy to unhealthy bacteria is off, or the toxins are moving too slow in the tract, some of the bacteria can end up being transformed to toxins and become reabsorbed. They therefore have to go back to the liver for reconversion.

A problem occurs when the two phases are not in sync. When enzymes of the liver operate at a different pace, for instance if the first one works faster than the second one, it lead to a buildup of toxic intermediate by products that can react and damage your DNA. The foods and drinks we consume and hormones we produce have a direct influence on the enzymes of the liver. This means that our diet can have a direct impact on how fast the enzymes move and either promote a toxic build up or promote a synchronized balance. We therefore need plenty of vitamins, enzymes and other molecules to help the body get rid of the waste products and toxins; hence, the need for our body to manufacture enzymes and molecules to help take the good from what we take in and get rid of the rest.

If the cell junctions within the small intestines are too tight, it becomes impossible for the large fat molecules to pass through cell wall into the lymphatic tissue. Consequently, these larger fat-soluble molecules move down the gut as bile follows it and absorbs the toxins that are fat soluble which are then eliminated along with stool thus making it to have a dark brown color. But if the bile doesn't bind to the toxins and the toxins are not eliminated along with the stool (especially when your meal is deficient of fiber), then your body recycles them (up to 94%) up into the liver (the bile along with the toxic buildup). If this happens over a long time, your liver can start getting overwhelmed since it is not usually expecting the return of various toxic fat cells. As more and more toxins and bile mixture gets recycled, this forms a thick and sludgy mixture, which may in turn make it hard for it to break down any fatty foods, along with fat soluble toxins. This may in even progress to a point where the bile becomes too thick and sluggish such that it cannot buffer the stomach acids that usually start entering the small intestines. Consequently, this acid starts acting as an irritant to the villi resulting to congestive reactive mucus production. And as the bile increasingly becomes viscous, it may end up blocking the flow of different pancreatic enzymes right into your small intestines. Keep in mind that your pancreas usually shares the same bile duct with the gallbladder so if the duct is blocked, this may affect other aspects of digestion.

Over time, the biliary tubes within the liver can become too congested with toxins and thick bile. In response, the liver starts pushing the fat soluble toxins into the bloodstream (probably to create room for more!). Unfortunately, these toxins are harmful to different body organs so the body has to find a way of 'protecting' its vital organs from damage by toxins. In response, it pushes these fat soluble toxins into the fat cells where they are stored 'safely' for years.

Unfortunately, with continuous toxicity, this results to build up of more fat in order to store the growing toxicity. And as a result, you will end up gaining weight rapidly as your body rapidly figures a way of protecting its vital organs and systems from toxins. This means that your body cannot just burn the fat that it is using to protect you from toxins since doing so will mean releasing harmful substances into circulation, which means this type of fat is very hard to lose (it is mostly found around the belly). In addition, it means that you may find it impossible to lose weight until you detoxify no matter how little you eat.

However, just because the toxins are stored in fat cells away from 'vital' organs doesn't mean that they don't affect you in any way. They do; in fact, they cause such problems like oxidation (this simply means free radical damage) along with degeneration). In addition, some toxins may somehow find their way into the brain resulting to what is referred to as neurotoxicity, which is very dangerous given that it can cause cognitive problems and various other health imbalances.

With this understanding, it will be easier for you to understand how toxins cause other health complications.

2. Heart disease

Heart disease is the #1 killer in the US today accounting for more than half of all deaths annually (over

610,000). Diets high in saturated fats and cholesterol, obesity, diabetes, excessive use of alcohol, and not getting enough exercise are the leading causes of heart disease that you may probably know of. Several chemicals have also been linked to the heart disease, like arsenic in drinking water. Studies estimate that for every 15mg/L increase in arsenic in your drinking water, this increases the risk of suffering from heart disease by 38%. Other toxins linked to heart disease include antimony, BPA and triclosan.

3. Cancer

The toxins in cigarettes have been linked to causing lung cancer. However, about 10% of lung cancer for non-smokers is due to exposure to toxins like radon, asbestos or diesel exhaust. According to the present statistics, 1 in 2 men or 1 in 3 women that will get cancer in their lifetime will be as a result of exposure to toxins. Some of the toxins with strongest links to cancer include:

• The nitrates and iron in red and processed meat have been linked to lung, gastric, bladder, colorectal and esophageal cancer.

• Arsenic and byproducts of water disinfection that are found in your drinking water are linked to bladder cancer.

• Many pesticides like atrazine have been linked to breast and prostate cancer.

• Endocrine disrupters like BPA and parabens have been linked to breast and prostate cancer.

4. Diabetes

Type 2 diabetes is a disease whereby your body cannot make good use its own insulin or it does not make enough insulin in the first place. This results to excessive accumulation of glucose within your bloodstream. The hormone insulin (insulin is responsible for triggering the body cells to open up to absorb glucose from the bloodstream) is produced by pancreas, which is part of the endocrine system. This makes it a prime target for endocrine disrupting chemicals like BPA and other different types of pesticides. And just like for the case of cancer and heart disease, arsenic in water has a hand in causing diabetes.

5. Parkinson's disease

This is the second most common neurodegenerative disorder. Only 5% of the cases are hereditary while the remaining 95% is linked to toxins and severe head injuries. Pesticides seem to have the strongest link of all the toxins believed to cause PD. Any chemical that is a neurotoxin can affect your brain and nervous system (we mentioned that toxins can find their way into your brain). Pesticides are good example of a neurotoxin. Specific pesticides linked to PD are insecticides.

Obviously, these potential risks of increased toxicity within your body should give you enough motivation to want to take action. But to give you even a greater boost, let me show you some reasons why you should detoxify.

Why We Need to Detox

1. To remove toxins from the body

The long-term exposure to toxins affects our behavior, metabolism and immune system leading to various diseases- I mentioned some of these diseases in the previous chapter.

2. To prevent chronic diseases

Increased build up of toxins within your body exposes you to the risk of many chronic diseases such as cancer, stokes, heart diseases, neurological disorders...you name them. Because our built-in detox functions are always overloaded, detoxing assists in improving what our bodies try to do naturally.

3. Lose weight

Toxins rid our body of our natural ability to burn fats leading to weight gain. I mentioned that your body uses fat cells to bind toxins to keep them off circulation and from various vital organs. Unfortunately, as you accumulate more fat to bind toxins, you end up gaining weight, which is a risk factor to such health complications as high blood pressure, diabetes and heart diseases. By detoxing, you free the fat cells that had toxins of what they were holding, which in turn means that you end up making it possible for you to burn this fat (remember you cannot burn the toxin filled fats!). As a result, losing weight (especially belly fat) becomes a lot easier for you.

4. To enhance the immune system

Toxins make us vulnerable to colds and flu, which as you well know affect our productivity and quality of life by weakening our immune system. Detoxing regularly helps strengthen the functioning of our immune system thus making it easier for us to fight infection.

5. To improve the quality of life

Some of the symptoms that come with increased toxin build up within your body include extreme fatigue, headaches, sleep problems and even digestive disorders. Detoxification can ease depression and improve your memory besides solving all the listed problems. You will also have more physical, emotional and mental energy. You will also tend to have a good night sleep without the need to oversleep!

6. Improve the quality of the skin

What we eat and the toxins within our environment majorly affect our skin. When we have high levels of toxicity, this is likely to show through dull skin, acne breakouts, uneven skin tone, rashes, itching and other symptoms. The good news is that detoxing gives us a natural healthy glow by improving acne and strengthening our hair and nails.

7. Restores a balance to our body's system

Our nervous, digestive and hormonal systems were designed to work together for optimal health achievement. When we keep overloading our bodies with toxins and the wrong kinds of foods, it becomes hard to achieve this unity, which results to us being sick. Detoxing brings back the balance and helps the systems function together again.

8. To improve mental and emotional clarity

When our body systems are well aligned and working properly, a shift occurs to our mental and emotional states. When we are mentally and emotionally clear, we can make better decisions, are likely to make better analysis and usually tend to see stuff from a better perspective.

The good news is that exposure to toxins is not a guarantee that you are going to be sick especially because diseases are usually caused by a combination of things including genetics and your lifestyle besides toxins exposure. However, this doesn't mean that you should do nothing about the situation - you can do nothing about your genes but you can manipulate your lifestyle and your exposure to toxins to stay safe! The truth is that there is a lot you can do to transform your body's toxicity.

To get us started, let's learn some simple yet effective ways on how to reduce our exposure to toxins and boost your body's natural detox process:

Natural Ways of reducing toxic load

1. Use chemical-free cosmetics, cleaning products and body care. This might sound impossible in this century but there are many companies that are making chemical free products.

2. Find your toxic triggers. You know your body better so you can easily tell what works for you and what doesn't. Toxins could build up from foods that react with your body and cause you allergies. Once you know your triggers, stay away from it.

3. Avoid overconsumption of alcohol and pills. Too much alcohol consumption can damage your liver just like some certain drugs. A damaged liver is difficult to reverse- almost impossible.

4. Get moving. This helps your blood and the lymphatic system to do its job. This will improve the general detoxing process.

5. Eat whole foods and non-GMO. The major source of chemicals and toxins come from the foods we eat. Look for whole foods that are free from preservatives, conservatives and coloring agents. Choose chemical free and organic varieties if they are available. Besides taking whole foods and non-GMO, it is also critical that

you supercharge the detox process by taking specific foods/drinks that fasten the process. One such food/drink is tea. The rest of this book will focus using tea to detox.

Tea For Detox

We all know how important regular detoxing is when it comes to removing toxins from our body. Detoxing doesn't have to be an occasional thing; we can do it almost every single day by avoiding chemically laden foods and eating organic foods. Another way to help detox on a daily basis is by drinking certain teas especially because the potent power of tea is known worldwide- drinking detoxifying teas with high antioxidant cleansing powers can help you gain high detoxing powers and help you remove the harmful substances that have made your body their home. The teas aim to help with the cleansing process, strengthening and toning your organs and finally eliminate toxins from your body. So which teas should you take to detox?

Best Teas For Detox

1. Red clover Tea

Red clover comes full of anti-oxidant compounds that give your body serious back up when it comes to killing the free radicals that cause diseases. It can also help you to build strength from the inside. It is a diaphoretic, which means that it stimulates sweating, which in turn helps get rid of toxins through the skin. The flowers are the part of the plant that helps with cleansing purposes. Red clover flower can last for up to a year when dried up.

The Chinese used this tea traditionally to remove toxins from the liver and the blood. It stimulates the production of bile that helps the liver to process fats in your body. The anti-inflammatory properties of the red clover also helps prevent the inflammation of the liver and thus improving on its efficiency.

You can use the flower to clear the lungs of phlegm and toxins for it is an excellent expectorant. Additionally, red clover is rich in vitamins B and C thus making it highly nutritious.

To make strong red clover tea, use ½ cup of dried flowers in 3 cups of hot water. Add a pinch of mint, steep for two hours then reheat and strain. Drink a cup after each of the three main meals.

2. Burdock Tea

This herb has been used for years for blood purification purposes. Burdock tea has powerful detoxifying benefits because its root is a powerful diuretic so through urine, it helps your body purge out toxins.

Additionally, this herb contains an organic compound referred to as polyacetylene, which is rich in antifungal and antibacterial properties that not only cleanse the blood but also stimulates the immune system.

In addition, burdock root is a diaphoretic, which means that it has the ability to promote sweating, which in turn helps to remove toxins through the skin.

It also treats acne, as it increases the circulation of blood under the skin and helps detoxify the epidermal tissues of your body.

Increased removal of toxins from the body aids the liver because it lessens the amount of toxins re-introduced back to your bloodstream to compromise the functioning of the liver.

Ensure to select burdock roots carefully ensuring that you use the one that is firm and not too soft. Clean the root and then chop coarsely about 2 tablespoons of its root then place it in a small stainless pot then proceed to add 3 cups of water and bring to a boil. Then lower the heat then simmer for 3o minutes. Allow to steep for another 20 minutes then serve hot. Drink it throughout the day as detox tea.

3. Ginger Tea

Ginger tea is a superior cleansing root when brewed. The good thing is that ginger is very gentle on your body, even though it might be too strong for your taste buds. So how does it help in detox?

Well, ginger helps cleanse your body by stimulating digestion, improving blood circulation and improving the efficiency with which you sweat (which essentially means you will be removing more toxins).

It is also great at removing a buildup of wastes and toxins in the colon and liver.

You can make this detox tea each morning, in the afternoon or as a warm up after dinner.

4. Cayenne pepper tea

You can always brew this spice as tea or add it directly into your diet.

Cayenne pepper stimulates your circulation system by opening up capillaries, regulating your blood sugar and helping with your digestion. It is a great way to kick-start your metabolism for the energy you are going to use all day.

It can make you detox your body by removing more toxins through your mucus and phlegm. In addition, it is a natural antiviral and antifungal spice, which should protect you against colds and flus. Try drinking some hot lemon juice with 1/8 teaspoon of cayenne pepper to detox every morning.

5. Dandelion tea

Dandelion tea raises the amount of enzymes in the liver that are responsible for detox. It supports and stimulates the functioning of the liver and helps to improve the functioning of the gall bladder in the production of bile, which is an essential ingredient in the detoxing process. This tea should be one you should consider adding to your diet because it also helps remove carcinogens (these are substances known to cause cancer).

It is also a great diuretic since it helps you remove more toxins through urination.

Additionally, it is perfect for cleaning your digestive tract. A cup of dandelion tea on an empty stomach every morning will cleanse your alimentary canal, stop constipation, GERD and any other problem with digestion.

Dandelion tea also prevents kidney stones and gallbladder stones. It can also cleanse your skin from inside out as it hiders the growth of bacteria.

You can make your own dandelion tea from its roots or flowers. Steep the flowers or roots in boiling water then proceed to strain the flowers and the roots. 2-3 cups a day are enough.

6. Fenugreek tea

This tea is made from seeds of the fenugreek plant.

The good thing about it is that it helps lower blood pressure, reduce inflammation and support the ability of your liver to remove toxins from your body.

The tea is also known to regulate blood sugar levels by slowing the rate at which the sugar enters your blood stream.

Fenugreek tea is also a laxative that makes it a great way of removing toxins from your body through the bowels. As such, drinking fenugreek tea on a daily basis is therefore a great way to help keep body clean.

Another way it will remove toxins from your body is through the skin. If you experience a strong perspiration smell, it could be the result of an unhealthy diet as the tea eliminates the dirt.

Use whole fenugreek seeds to make your own tea. Use about 1 teaspoon of fenugreek seeds to make a cup. Soak the seeds in boiling water for 15 minutes then let it sit for another few minutes before you strain and drink. 2-3 cups a day is enough but you can drink as much as you like to enjoy the health benefits.

7. Fennel tea

Fennel tea is made from the Mediterranean plant Foeniculum vulgar, which is a member of the carrot family. The tea is made from the plant's seeds, which you can easily confuse with anise.

A cup of fennel herbal tea is rich in vitamins A, B-complex, C and D and antioxidants not forgetting that it is a great source of amino acids.

Fennel tea eliminates toxins from your body through urine because it is a diuretic. Additionally, it helps increase the healthy flow of urine within the respective organs as well as helps to protect the liver against damage from alcohol. It also has the ability to treat diseases like jaundice.

The vitamins improve the functioning of the kidney and prevent kidney stones. In addition, it helps reduce the retention of water making it one of the best weight loss teas for you, since it also helps you to burn fats faster and reduce cellulite.

By using this healthy tea to cleanse your body, you improve the health of your joints and tissues thus relieving gout and other arthritic pains.

Besides detoxing, fennel tea also promotes a strong heart, improves your hormonal balance, treat your eyes of infection like conjuvities and above all, improves your digestion.

To take fennel tea, take 1 teaspoon of dried fennel seeds per cup of tea and pour hot water over it. Boiling the seeds kills most of its nutrients so don't boil them;

simply cover it and let it rest for 10 minutes. You will get a yellow infusion- drink it 3 times a day. The best time to take it is after meals so as to also help with digestion problems.

8. Chinese teas

These teas can be categorized into 5 different groups: Black tea, green tea, white tea, oolong tea and post fermented tea. They all come from the leaves of camellia sinensis plant. The difference arises due to the differences in processing methods, the geographical location from where the tea plant was grown along with the appearance and the taste of the infused tea. The various variations also bring out the difference in the amount of chlorophyll present in each variety.

When you drink Chinese teas, the chlorophyll in it attaches itself to the toxins and heavy metals in the body. Chlorophyll is rich in anti-inflammatory along with antioxidant properties that usually contribute to its great cleansing effects.

By stimulating the production of red blood cells, chlorophyll increases the carrying capacity of oxygen in your blood. This can in turn boost your lung's detoxing ability.

Besides cleansing the blood, chlorophyll has the ability to cleanse the liver, thanks to its ability to prevent substances that cause cancer from attaching to the cells.

The magnesium content in chlorophyll also helps to promote the healthy functioning of your immune system and decrease stress, which in turn helps to prevent toxins from accumulating within your body by simply providing a great calming effect. The vitamins E, A and C in chlorophyll support your immune system by strengthening the walls of your cells and reducing oxidation, which is step one in defending against toxins for them.

Among the five groups, Green tea is the oldest and most popular type of tea. It is made from the tea plant's green shoots, which are then dried and processed according to the type of green tea you like. There are 4 different processing techniques for green tea including: sun-dried, roasted, stir-fried and steamed. Traditionally, green tea has a pale color and a sharp astringent flavor. It also has the highest amount of chlorophyll

Green tea is an excellent source of antioxidants called polyphenols. These antioxidants play a role in treating and preventing a variety of health conditions; of the most potent of these antioxidant compounds is EGCG. The possible detoxifying effects of the polyphenols including EGCG in green tea come from their role in helping your body eliminate free radicals, which can otherwise damage healthy cells. The antioxidant properties of EGCG might play some role in helping to prevent diverse conditions such as genital warts, liver disease, bacterial infections and different types of cancer including breast, prostate and colorectal cancer.

2 to 3 cups of green are enough in a day to get you about 240 to 320 mg of polyphenols. The best way to make sure you are getting the most out of it is by making it yourself because pre-made green tea has far less natural value. In any case, brewing and drinking of green tea is a beautiful and calming ritual. Moreover, the leftovers of green tea leaves have dozens of other uses.

There are literally countless versions of green tea. The difference emerges from the different locations of where they are grown, a slight change in their cultivation and the different climate in the different locations (for instance, in Japan, we have bancha, sencha, gyokuro, gemaicha, kukicha, houjicha and matcha).

Matcha Green Tea

Although tea was first discovered in China and became part of its tradition, it also became an important part of the Japanese culture. They named their tea "matcha". This tea is commonly used in Japanese tea ceremony. In fact, the Zen Buddhist monks usually drink it when they want to remain calm and alert when meditating for long hours.

The Japanese grow their tea in the shade to increase the chlorophyll content. The shade ensures the chlorophyll remains extant instead of being converted by sunlight into catechins. These chlorophyll-rich leaves are then hand-picked and then stone-ground into fine powder. Matcha is therefore a special type of powdered green tea. It does not look or taste likes other kinds of tea. It looks like electric green cocoa and has a mouth-feel of a well-made espresso. The high level of chlorophyll is what it uses to remove heavy metals such as lead, mercury and cadmium and other harmful chemicals from the body. The chlorophyll also de-acidifies the body and restores its natural PH balance as well as cleans and purifies the blood.

When you brew a cup of green tea, you end up throwing valuable minerals and antioxidants after water only extracting a fraction of the teas benefits. The remaining antioxidants get trapped in the tea leaves, unused. The one way to take advantage of the green tea leaves is by consuming the entire leaf not by eating the tea leaves, but by simply enjoying a bowl of matcha. Matcha provides you fully with vitamins, minerals, and amino acids in its special way, which makes it more like whole food than tea. In fact the potency found in a single serving of matcha equals approximately 10 cups of brewed green tea.

Matcha is an antioxidant powerhouse; it has 6.2 times more the level of antioxidants found in Goji Berries, 17 times more than that in wild blueberries, 7 times the amount in dark chocolate and 60.5 times that of spinach. Antioxidants are naturally occurring chemical compounds that prevent aging and chronic diseases. The more you have, the more your body is equipped to fight against infections and diseases.

Because of the amino-acid l-thiamine present in it, matcha will enhance your moods by helping alleviate both anxiety and depression without the jittery and negative aspects of coffee or energy drinks. Matcha has roughly 25 mg of caffeine per serving, which is way less than the amount in brewed coffee, usually about 8o-100 mg per serving. Additionally, the caffeine in matcha is not acidic; it is alkalizing. This property makes it much gentler in our stomach hence making it perfect for cleansing and improved digestion. To add on that, the caffeine in matcha tends to act as 'timed release.' It is therefore absorbed into your bloodstream at a much slower rate than the case with coffee.

The quality of matcha tea

Unlike normal tealeaves, it is very easy to tell good matcha from bad matcha. Color is the biggest factor while accessing the quality of matcha. In particular, you can tell by simply looking at it. Quality matcha should be electric green or bright green while bad matcha will be a dull green, army green or even yellowish in the worst case. These colors are not a good sign. It could mean several things:

• It could mean that the matcha contains stems and branches

• It could be that the matcha is well past its prime

• A combination of the first two cases

The aroma also comes in as another quality assessment factor. Your matcha should smell fresh, inviting and vegetal. If it does smell a bit stale like old hay, you don't have the best quality of matcha with you.

How to prepare matcha green tea in four easy steps

1. Sift 2 tablespoons matcha into a cup using a small sieve.

2. Boil 2 ounces of water to about 85 degrees C and add it to your cup.

3. In a zigzag motion, whisk vigorously until the tea is frothy.

4. Enjoy your matcha.

Benefits Of Drinking Green Tea Over Coffee

1. Green tea contains flavonoids

Matcha contains polyphenols such as flavonoids and catechins. Catechins are a class of powerful antioxidants that are known to prevent cell damage. Generally, antioxidants are good at having positive effects on your general health. Consider adding antioxidants to your diet to slow down aging in addition to your other anti-aging strategies. To get the most catechins from matcha green tea, use water that is quite not yet to boiling point; too hot water destroys the antioxidants in the powder.

Coffee does not contain any catechins, a good reason why you should replace your morning coffee with a cup of green matcha tea with a squeeze of lemon. Lemon contains vitamin C that will help catechins to be absorbed more efficiently. Choose from a higher quality brand of green tea because some of the lower quality brands could contain excessive levels of fluoride.

2. Green tea lowers bad cholesterol levels

Besides improving your general cellular health, catechins have the power to reduce harmful cholesterol and increase good cholesterol. When the ratio of bad to good cholesterol is high, it means that you are at a great risk of having a heart attack or worse, a stroke. Green tea increases the oxidant capability of the blood, which protects the LD cholesterol particles from oxidation, which is one of the pathways towards heart diseases. Drinking more coffee raises your bad cholesterol levels unlike when you enjoy a cup of matcha. Switching to matcha in conjunction with a good diet and exercise will help you reduce the cholesterol levels and maintain a good and healthy heart.

3. Matcha is great for the mind

Because green tea helps you out so much with the health of your heart, the result is healthier blood vessels in your brain and improved mental clarity. Green tea also improves your general cognitive function. Caffeine is a known stimulant. Coffee contains a lot of it but the little that the green tea has is enough to produce response without jittery and other negative responses of coffee. What the caffeine does in the brain is that it blocks an inhibitory neurotransmitter referred to as adenosine. This way, it increases the firing neurons and the concentration of neurotransmitters such as dopamine.

Green tea contains more than just caffeine. It is also rich in l- theanine, an amino acid, which has been proven to have the ability to cross the brain barrier. L-theanine usually increases the activity of GABA, an inhibitory neurotransmitter, which has anti-anxiety effects. It also increases alpha and dopamine wave production in the brain. With a very high amount of caffeine, coffee puts you at two times the risk of developing cognitive impairment when you drink it daily. Matcha green tea is the solution to powerful long -term health benefits.

4. Matcha has healthier caffeine

The high caffeine content in coffee causes a number of unpleasant side effects. This includes a rapid heartbeat, twitching, irritability, nausea, anxiety, headaches and many others. Coffee may taste delicious but interestingly, Matcha green tea has less than a quarter of the caffeine content that's found in coffee. The green tea also has a slow release of the caffeine into the digestive tract (and the brain) unlike the coffee, which releases its caffeine at a go. If you want a slight energy boost while avoiding the many downsides that come with drinking too much caffeine, you should try taking a cup of matcha tea every morning. The less caffeine also mean better good night sleep and your sleep schedule will slowly graduate to a normal healthy pattern.

5. Green tea helps in managing diabetes

Studies have revealed that if you are a diabetic who drinks coffee, you have a hard time regulating your blood sugar. Type II diabetes involves the inability of your body to produce insulin or having elevated blood sugar levels coupled with insulin resistance. Studies have revealed that green tea helps regulate type II diabetes by indirectly preventing dietary sugar from being metabolized. From this, unsweetened matcha then remains the great option to replace your daily coffee with because it also lowers the risk of developing type II diabetes in the long run.

6. Green tea increases your metabolism

Compared to coffee, matcha still tastes great without sugar. For many of us, we will find it hard to drink a cup of coffee without sugar and or milk. By switching to drink matcha green tea instead of coffee, you save yourself from tons of empty calories and still lose weight faster. There is also evidence that with green tea, you will lose weight faster by increasing your fat burning rate and speeding up your metabolism.

7. Matcha improves your mood

Apart from catechins, matcha green tea contains an amino acid called theanine, a powerful mood booster. It increases your levels of serotonin, dopamine, chemicals that are important in transforming your mood (they are feel good hormones). It also improves blood pressure, anxiety and mental clarity. If you are struggling with anxiety and depression, then matcha is the sure way to go as theanine will help ease these symptoms. Coffee has no thiamine. Besides, it is known to increase anxiety.

8. Green tea may protect your brain in old age thus lowering the risk of Parkinson's and Alzheimer's

Green tea will not only improve your brain function in short term; it will also protect your brain in old age. It will prevent the neuro-degeneration of the brain that leads to Alzheimer's. Parkinson's disease is the second most common neurodegenerative disease that involves the death of dopamine producing neurons in your brain. L-thianine in green tea increases the production of the dopamine in the brain.

9. Matcha is simple to make

Matcha carries some practical benefit besides its health importance; it is quick and easy to make. Matcha green tea is finely ground powder, which means that instead of waiting for it to steep, you can dissolve it in hot water and drink it instantly. You don't have to stand there and watch it brew for 15 minutes or more like you would do with the coffee maker.

Here are some other benefits of green tea:

Weight Loss and green Tea

As we have seen earlier, green tea is more than just hot flavored water. Green tea can help you lose weight in quite a number of ways. First, for us to burn fats that make us gain weight, it must first be broken down in the fat cells and moved into the blood stream. The main antioxidant in green tea, EGCG can aid this process by boosting the effects of some fat burning hormones norepinephrine. The end result is that more fat cells break down more fat, which is released into the bloodstream and become available for use as energy by muscles that need it.

Second and finally, as green tea helps you detox, it automatically makes you take in fewer calories by reducing your appetite and reduces the amount of fat we absorb from food.

Rehydration

If your body lacks enough water, tea will help rehydrate it. Just like what water does to your body, when you detoxify with green tea, it will help purify your blood, flush out toxins, treat constipation and still enhance its digestive function.

Better Skin

How your skin looks like is a reflection of what is going on inside your body. If you have plenty of toxins, you will see it through your skin as rashes, cracks or sometimes a dry skin if you are dehydrated. Green tea has the power to restore the smooth texture of your skin because of the vitamins and all the nutrients it contains. If you have acne scars or you want to prevent them, use a green tea tonner. The tonner can also greatly reduce the acne induced inflammation and perfectly soothe your skin.

With that in mind, let's take a quick look at how to make different tasty tea recipes to lose weight, detox, boost your metabolism and a lot more.

Tea Cleanse Diet Recipes

Red Clover Tea Recipe

Yields: 4 servings

Ingredients

2 tablespoons mint

1 cup red clover blossoms

4 cups water

Honey to sweeten

Instructions

1. Inspect the red clover flowers and make sure there are no bugs. Make sure the flowers are not sprayed.

2. Bring the water to a boil and then remove from heat then proceed to add clover blossoms and mint then steep for about 10 minutes and strain. Add honey to taste and enjoy.

Burdock Tea Recipe

Yields: 10 servings

Ingredients

12 cups of water

Honey or stevia for sweetened

3-inch piece fresh ginger, peeled and thinly sliced

2 stalks lemongrass, woody ends trimmed and thinly sliced

2 burdock rots, peeled and roughly chopped

Instructions

1. Combine the lemongrass, burdock, ginger and water in a large stock pot.

2. Bring the mixture to a boil then reduce the heat and simmer while partially covered for 20 minutes.

3. Strain the mixture then sweeten with honey and enjoy.

Garlic Tea Recipe

Yields: 3 ½ cups

Ingredients

½ cup fresh lemon juice

½ cup honey

3 garlic cloves, cut in half

3 cups water

Instructions

1. Bring 3 cups of water and the 3 cloves of garlic to a boil in a saucepan then turn off the heat when the water boils and add ½ cup of the honey and ½ cup of fresh lemon juice.

2. Strain ½ cup of warm tea three times a day then refrigerate the extra to use the next day.

Green Fennel Seeds Tea

Yields: 1 serving

Ingredients

¾ teaspoon tea leaves

1 teaspoon sugar

¾ teaspoon fennel seed, crushed

1 ½ cups water

Instructions

1. Boil fennel seeds in water 3 minutes.

2. Add tealeaves, turn off heat and let the tea stand for a while.

3. Stir in the sugar and enjoy.

How To Make Green Tea

Yields: 1 serving

Ingredients

Honey to taste

1 cup water

1 teaspoon green tea leaves (available ready-made)

Instructions

1. Heat 1 cup of water but do not bring it to boil; switch it off before it boils.

2. Add 1 teaspoon of green tea and brew it for about 3 minutes.

3. Then strain the tea into a cup

4. Add honey and a few drops of lemon juice to taste. Enjoy it while it is still hot.

Fenugreek Tea Recipe

Yields: 2 servings

Ingredients

2 teaspoons fenugreek

2 cups water

Loose tea leaves

Instructions

1. Crush the seeds lightly using a pestle and motor.

2. Bring the two cups of water to a boil in a saucepan and then proceed to pour the boiled water into a teapot.

3. Add the crushed fenugreek seeds then add other loose tealeaves then cover and steep the seeds for at least 3 minutes.

4. Strain the tea into a cup then sweeten with sugar or honey if desired. Enjoy hot or cold.

Iced Lime Dandelion Tea

Yields: 8 servings

Ingredients

3 quarts cold water

1 quart fresh handpicked dandelion flowers

Juice from 4 limes

1 cup hot water (not quite boiling)

3 tablespoons dried stevia leaf or a sweetener of your own choice

½ cup dried raspberry leaf

Instructions

1. Rinse the fresh dandelions well with cold water and ensure they are not sprayed with pesticides.

2. In a cup, pour hot water over the stevia leaf and dried red raspberry leaf and then stir well. Let this steep for 8 minutes tops then strain off the herbs.

3. Pour the sweetened liquid (the one with stevia and raspberry) into a gallon-size glass jar then add the juice of lime and then the cool water.

4. Mix gently after adding the dandelion flowers. Refrigerate for at least 4 hours then strain the flowers out and enjoy the tea within 36 hours.

Honey-Lemon Ginger Tea Recipe

Yields: 4 cups

Ingredients

3 tablespoons of honey

2 lemons, juiced

3 teabags

¼ cup grated ginger root

¾ cup brown sugar

4 cups water

Instructions

1. Stir water, grated ginger root and brown sugar together in a saucepan then bring to boil and then reduce the heat to medium-low. Cook at a simmer for 20 minutes.

2. Remove the saucepan from the heat and add tea bags before you steep the tea for 5 minutes. Remove the teabags.

3. Then proceed to stir the lemon juice and honey into the tea and strain into a pitcher.

Cayenne Pepper Tea With Ginger

Yields: 4 servings

Ingredients

2 tablespoons lemon juice

½ teaspoon cayenne pepper

1 small ginger, peeled

4 cups water

A sweetener to taste

Instructions

1. Start by grating the ginger root into the water and then proceed to bring the water to a steady boil before you simmer for 10-15 minutes.

2. Next, add in the cayenne pepper before simmering for another 3 minutes then remove the tea from the heat, add lemon juice then stir and finally sweeten the tea.

Matcha Mint Iced Tea

Yields: 2 servings

Ingredients

A handful of mint

1 lime, sliced

2 cups crushed ice

2 teaspoons cooking grade matcha

2 cups filtered water

Honey to sweeten

Instructions

1. Shake together the matcha and the water using a cocktail shaker until there are no lumps. Then proceed to add the ice, the handful mint, a squeeze of lime and shake it some more. Add honey to sweeten.

2. Pour into glasses with mint and extra lime slices.

All this information may be a bit confusing when you just don't know how you can follow it in your day to day life. To make the process easy for you, let's discuss a 7 week plan on how to go about it.

An Easy to Follow 7 Day Tea Detox Plan

Day 1

Read about detoxing and know why you want to detox. Know the benefits of what you want to get yourself into. Make notes of important points if possible. They will act as a guide and a point of reference whenever you feel like you are out of track. Stay positive that what you are about to do is for your own good. If your goal is to have a smooth skin or to lose weight, I would advise you take a photo of you before you start to compare with the one you will take at the end of the 7 day program.

For this day, you will take 1 cup of Red Clover Tea (preferably as part of your breakfast) so simply refer to the recipes section above on how to make it.

Day 2

In your notebook, make a list of foods to avoid and what to eat. When you are starting your tea detox program, your diet will play an important part of your success. It is therefore important to know what type of food to eat. You won't have to drink concoctions that are absurd or live on tea and fruits alone. The best way to go about it is by simply eating healthy on top drinking all the natural green tea.

While on the program, it is important to eat a lot of fruits and vegetables because they are filled with macronutrients to fill your body. Pick the ones with vibrant colors like leafy green for vegetables, or any type of berries for fruits.

Avoid any enriched or white grains and opt for healthier and natural grain such as quinoa and brown rice. You will also want to stay away from any sugary, fatty, foods that are processed and alcohol as they contain the same toxins your body is trying to get rid of. In your notebook, make a list of natural and healthy foods in conjunction with your detoxing tea for the detoxing period to get maximum results by giving your body a chance to reset itself fully.

During this day, you can take 2 cups of Burdock Tea (refer to the recipes section) after breakfast and in your afternoon (after lunch) beverage.

Day 3

For day three, you can take a cup of matcha green tea three times a day i.e. before you eat your breakfast, lunch and dinners for a soothing and calming effect throughout your day. You will notice increased energy levels in the morning and a good night sleep with no bloating.

Day 4

Go for a morning jog. Exercising is also one of the ways of detoxing. Keep in mind that detoxing with tea alone will not grant you maximum results. Combining 'teatox' with a bit of exercise will give you excellent results.

Exercise will increase lymph flow and circulation to help you lose toxins by sweating. When you take a cup of fenugreek tea after the run, you will drive even more toxins out as fenugreek tea detoxes through the skin.

Day 5

Detox the mind. It is good to clear the clutter from your mind too as you clean your body. Even 5 minutes of meditation in a day will help detox your mind and hence your body. Meditation will improve your mental functioning, ease depression and reduce stress and anxiety. Meditation brings us back to the present moment and encourages better decision making. A clean body and clear mind allows us to experience our lives to the fullest. If you don't know how to go about it, here are a few easy steps on how to go about;

Step 1: Get to a comfortable place and breathe. If it's on a chair, sit upright with your back straight, your legs under your feet and your palms resting on your lap. Look straight ahead without necessarily focusing on anything. Start feeling your feet after taking a deep breath; feel them touching the ground and their surrounding temperature-do not think about them. Just sense them.

Step 2: Scan your body with attention. Take some more deep breathes and shift your attention from your feet slowly moving up; start with your thighs, then your abdomen, your back, your arms your neck, face and finally your head. Stop and take deep breaths for every part of your body you scan. This practice will straighten your ability to hold and direct your attention.

Step 3: Acknowledge your thoughts without judging them. While you are trying to focus, thoughts will come and try to steal your attention. This is normal when you become aware of your baseline state. Becoming aware of this baseline state is the first step towards dissolving it and claiming back the energy it consumes. Then anchor your attention into the present as much as you can.

Step 4: Use this technique anywhere anytime you feel stressed. Practicing being present will help you clear your mind of quantum toxins and it will help you to stay more productive.

For this day, you can take matcha tea in the morning just before breakfast, Iced Lime Dandelion Tea just before lunch and Green Fennel Seeds Tea at night just before you've had dinner.

Day 6

Drink a cup of honey-lemon-ginger tea after your main meals. This is a good way to boost your digestion and cleanse your system at the same time.

Day 7

Chew your food properly before swallowing. Repeat steps 3, 4, 5 and 6 and note down their experiences and how they make you feel. Check out yourself in the mirror to see if there are any changes as compared to when you started the program. And do not forget to drink plenty of water during the entire detox plan. Three liters of fluid daily will help move the lymph and support kidney detoxification.

Note: As a rule of thumb, ensure to increase your fiber intake throughout this period. As such, your meals should include more of green leafy vegetables, cruciferous vegetables, fruits and anything else that is rich in natural fiber.

Note: Do not detox if you are breastfeeding, pregnant, underweight, elderly or have high blood pressure unless you have consulted with your medical practitioner.

Lavender Green Tea

1 ½ teaspoon Dried Lavender

2 teaspoons Green Tea

8 ounces of Water

Boil water. Put the lavender in an infuser and pour the boiling water over it. Let the lavender steep for 10 minutes. Add the green tea and steep for 2 to 3 minutes. If necessary, strain the water. You can allow the mixture to cool or drink it warm.

Cranberry Spritzer Green Tea

1/3 ounces of Water

4 teaspoons Green Tea

3 cups Seltzer

½ cup Cranberry Juice

Boil the water. Steep the 4 teaspoons of green tea for 2 to 3 minutes. Allow the mixture to cool then add the Seltzer and cranberry juice. If necessary, add honey to sweeten the mixture.

Kiwi and Mango Smoothie Green Tea

2 cups fresh Mango

¾ cup Vanilla Yogurt

½ teaspoon Lime Rind

3 Kiwis

½ cup Baby Spinach

2 teaspoons Loose Leaf Green Tea

2 tablespoons of Water

2 cups of Ice

Add all of the ingredients into a blender. If you prefer you can steep the green tea first in water and remove the leaves; however, you can also eat the leaves for their weight loss properties. Serve the drink after it is blended.

Almond and Blueberry Smoothie Green Tea

2 cups Fresh Blueberries

12 ounces Vanilla Yogurt

2 tablespoons Almonds

2 teaspoons Green Tea

2 tablespoons Flax Seeds

¾ cups Water

3 cups Ice

Boil the water and steep the green tea for 3 minutes. Put the tea infused water, plus all other ingredients into a blender and blend until smooth.

Rose Petal Green Tea

1 teaspoon Green Tea

1 Orange

1 teaspoon dried Rose and Hibiscus Petals

Remove the rind from the orange with a vegetable peeler. Let the rinds dry for one day before grinding them into a fine powder. Place the rind, green tea, and flowers into boiling water. Steep the mixture for 10 minutes, strain the mixture, and drink. You can also elect to drink this mixture cold. Depending on the sweetness of the orange, you may need to add a sweetener such as a dab of honey.

Tulsi Green Tea

1 teaspoon Green Tea

8 to 10 Tulsi Leaves

Honey (optional)

Chop the tulsi leaves then combine with the loose leaf green tea. Boil water. Pour the water over the tea infuser filled with the tea mixture. Let the combination steep for 3 to 4 minutes. Take out the tea infuser, add honey and serve. This green tea can also be served cold.

Minty Green Tea

2 teaspoons Green Tea

½ cup Fresh Mint Leaves

1 teaspoon Raw Honey

Wash and chop the fresh mint leaves, while the kettle water comes to a boil. Combine the tea and mint into a tea infuser. Pour the hot water over the mixture and allow it to steep for 3 to 4 minutes. You can serve this as an iced tea after 3 to 4 hours in the fridge, or serve right away. Add the honey just before serving.

Peach Mango White Tea

12 cups Water

5 teaspoons White Tea

2 Peaches

1 cup Mango

1 tablespoon Sugar, Rock Sugar, or Raw Honey

Boil the water. While the water is on the stove, take the time to remove the pits from the peaches and then dice the peaches and mangos. Steep the fruit and tea for 10 minutes. Add in the sweetening agent and serve. You can also serve this beverage cold. If you want to serve it cold, steep the white tea only. Remove the tea infuser, add the fruit, and allow the tea infused water and fruit to chill for 4 hours or a full day.

Thai Coconut Tea

2 cups Boiling Water

2 teaspoons Oolong Tea

1 cup Coconut Milk

1 Lemon Wedge

Fresh Mint, for garnish

Add the tea to the boiling water and steep for 3 minutes. Let the mixture cool, then add the milk, squeeze the lemon wedge and drop it into the tea, and garnish with a sprig of mint.

Grapefruit Oolong Tea

1 Red or Pink Grapefruit

½ cup Oolong Tea

1 drop Orange Bitters

1 teaspoon Raw Honey

Steep the Oolong tea into 4 cups of water for 5 minutes. Add the grapefruit slices, and orange bitters. Use honey or another sweetener. Let the mixture cool in the fridge for 4 hours.

Vitamin C Tisane

1 tablespoon Lemongrass

4 tablespoons Rose Hips

1 tablespoon Cinnamon Chips

1 teaspoon Fennel Seed

1 teaspoon Hibiscus Flowers

½ teaspoon Lemon Peel

4 cups Water

Fresh Fruit Juice (optional)

Combine all the herbs into an air tight container. When you want the tisane, boil 1 to 4 cups of water, adding in 1 to 4 teaspoons of the herb mixture to steep. Steep the mixture for 45 minutes. Add the fruit juice to sweeten the tisane. The Vitamin C Tisane can be served cold or hot, it is up to your tastes. All ingredients are high in Vitamin C, which is an essential nutrient for your health.

Honeycrisp Apple Black Tea

1 Honeycrisp Apple

½ cup Loose Leaf Black Tea

2 tablespoons Lemon Juice

15 Whole Cloves, chopped

2 Cinnamon Sticks, chopped

Sugar or Honey (optional)

Slice the apples as thinly as possible. Put the apples in a bowl with the lemon juice, cloves, and cinnamon for 5 minutes. Pre heat the oven to 350 degrees Fahrenheit. Bake the apples for 90 minutes. Allow the apples to dry and cool before chopping them finely. Combine with the tea into an air tight container. Whenever you want a cup of tea, use 1 teaspoon of the apple and black tea mixture to 8 ounces of water. Brew for 3 minutes.

After Dinner Digestive Tisane

1 teaspoon Spearmint Leaves

1/8 teaspoon Dried Licorice Root

1/8 Fennel Seeds

Combine the ingredients into an air tight container. Take one teaspoon to 8 ounces of boiled water, steep for 5 minutes, and then drink. The ingredients help aid in digestion by reducing gas and that full feeling you have. They also increase the metabolism. This tisane is best served hot, with a small dab of honey to sweeten it.

Tummy Taming Tisane

1/3 cup Calendula

¼ cup Fennel

¼ cup Marshmallow Root

½ cup Chamomile

Make sure all the ingredients are dried and finely chopped. Combine in an air tight container. When you need a digestive to reduce gas, bloating, or uncomfortable feelings in your tummy, brew 1 teaspoon of the tisane with 8 ounces of water. Calendula is known to help heal the intestinal lining of the stomach and reduce inflammation. Fennel helps calm the intestines, while marshmallow root can help sooth irritation for the stomach. It helps alleviate issues with the mucous membrane that covers the stomach and digestive tract, lessening issues with acid reflux and stomach ulcers. Chamomile is also an anti-inflammatory, and known to help relax a person's nerves.

Rejuvenating Goji Ginger White Tea

1 teaspoon Lemon Myrtle

2 tablespoons Dried Goji Berries

1 tablespoon Honeybush

1 teaspoon Dried Ginger Root

1 teaspoon Fennel Seeds

1 teaspoon Lemon Grass

2 tablespoons White Tea

Chop and dry the ingredients if they are not already in this condition. Combine all ingredients into an air tight jar. When you want a cup of tea, place 1 teaspoon of the mixture into a tea infuser, and pour 8 ounces of boiling water into the cup or teapot. Steep the tea infusion for 4 minutes.

Nettle Cinnamon White Tea

2 teaspoons Nettle

2 teaspoons Rose Hips

1 teaspoon Cinnamon Chips

2 tablespoons White Tea

4 cups Water

Raw Honey (optional)

In a medium mixing bowl combine the ingredients. Store the mixture in an air tight container. To brew the tea, use 1 teaspoon tea mixture and 8 ounces of boiling water. Steep the mixture for 4 to 5 minutes. Add the honey to sweeten the tea, if you wish.

Jack Frost Tisane

¼ cup Dried Spearmint Leaves

¼ cup Dried Peppermint Leaves

Combine the two ingredients into an air tight container. When you are ready to brew the tea to help with indigestion, nerves, headaches, or bloating put 1 teaspoon into a tea infuser. Boil 8 ounces of water then pour it over the tisane mixture. Allow it to steep for 5 to 15 minutes. If you like a strong mint flavor, you will want to steep the mixture longer.

Rosy Black Tea

2 teaspoons Rose Petals, dried

1 teaspoon Loose Leaf Black Tea

Combine the dried ingredients into an air tight mason jar. Shake until the ingredients are mixed. To prepare the tea, boil 8 ounces of water and pour over 1 teaspoon of the tea mixture. Steep the tea leaves and rose petals for 2 to 3 minutes. If you steep it longer the tea will become astringent.

Autumn Tonic White Tea

4 teaspoons Dried Nettle Leaf

3 teaspoons Lemon Balm

3 teaspoons Dried Spearmint Leaves

2 teaspoons Mullein Leaves

2 teaspoons Red Clover, chopped

2 teaspoons Dandelion Leaf and Root, dried

1 teaspoon Rose Hips

1 teaspoon Ginger Root, dried and chopped

4 teaspoons White Tea

Combine all of the ingredients into a bowl, mix thoroughly, and store in an air tight container.

To brew the mixture: place 1 teaspoon of the tea and herbs into a tea infuser. Boil 8 ounces of water and pour it into the mug with the infuser. Steep for 5 to 10 minutes, depending on how strong you like your tea.

Lavender Ruby Fruit Lemonade

6 Lemons, juiced

1 teaspoon Lavender

1 teaspoon Ruby Fruit

1/3 cup Sugar

Boil 2 cups of water, steep the lavender and ruby fruit for 15 minutes, strain, and pour into a one gallon container. Add the sugar and stir until dissolved. Add in the lemon juice then add water until the container is full.

Iced Green Tea with Lavender

Prepared with lavender blossoms, this chilled green tea mixture provides a subtle flavor. You can get lavender blossoms from your local health food store. This recipe makes one serving.

Ingredients:

-2 teaspoons of dried green tea leaves

-1 1/2 teaspoons of dried lavender blossoms

Directions:

1.Boil a cup of water in a kettle. Let it sit for a few minutes and allow it to cool a bit.

2.Put the dried tea leaves and dried lavender blossoms into the heated water. Allow it to steep for 3 to 5 minutes.

3.Strain the mixture and pour it in a glass with ice cubes.

*You may also stir in a teaspoon of honey for a sweeter blend.

Peachy Green Tea

Peach is referred to as the "Fruit of Calmness." That's because it helps you cope with stress and relieve anxiety. More than adding a refreshingly fruity flavor to your green tea, peach is an excellent source of phytochemicals, which aid in preventing weight problems related to heart diseases and diabetes. Moreover, this amazing concoction can make your skin glow. This recipe makes one serving.

Ingredients:

-1 cup of peeled and sliced peaches

-1 to 2 teaspoons of dried green tea leaves

Directions:

1.Boil water in a kettle. Let it sit for a few minutes and allow it to cool a bit.

2.Put the dried tea leaves in a cup and pour the heated water over it. Allow it to steep for 3 to 5 minutes.

3.In the meantime, pour a cup of the heated water in a saucepan over low flame. Add the peaches.

4.Stir continuously for 10 minutes. Set it aside.

5.Strain the green tea leaves.

6.Pour the green tea and peach mixture in a tall glass. Place it in the fridge for at least an hour.

7.Strain the mixture and add ice cubes for an even more refreshing drink.

Refreshing Green Tea with Melon

Melon contains weight loss properties too. This combination is a double threat against weight problems. It is also an effective drink for maintaining a youthful glow! This recipe makes one serving.

Ingredients:

-4 teaspoons of chopped mint tea leaves

-1/2 cup of melon slices

-1 to 2 teaspoons of dried green tea leaves

Directions:

1.Boil 2 cups of water in a kettle. Let it sit for a few minutes and allow it to cool a bit.

2.Put the dried tea leaves in a cup and pour the heated water over it. Allow it to steep for 3 to 5 minutes and strain.

3.Pour half of the heated water in a saucepan over medium heat.

4.Add the melon slices and chopped mint leaves.

5.Stir occasionally until the melon becomes tender. Set it aside to cool.

6.Pour the green tea and melon mixture into a glass. Stir and keep it in the fridge for about 2 hours.

7.Strain the mixture and enjoy!

Raspberry-licious Green Tea

Raspberries are a staple ingredient in weight loss juicing recipes. These juicy reds are not only rich on vitamins A, C and E. They are amazing for losing weight because of their Xylitol content, which is an excellent sugar substitute, but at low calories. This recipe makes one serving.

Ingredients:

-1 cup of fresh or frozen raspberries

-1 to 2 teaspoons of dried green tea leaves

Directions:

1.Boil 2 cups of water in a kettle. Let it sit for a few minutes and allow it to cool a bit.

2.Put the dried tea leaves in a cup and pour the heated water over it. Allow it to steep for 3 to 5 minutes and strain.

3.Pour half of the heated water in a saucepan over medium heat.

4.Add the raspberries into the pan and cook them until they are soft and start to break up. Set it aside to cool.

5.Pour the green tea and raspberry mixture in a glass. Stir and keep it in the fridge for about an hour.

6.Strain the mixture and stir. Bottoms up!

Green Tulsi Cleansing Tea

A great source of antioxidants, this powerful combination of green tea and tulsi leaves, provide an effective protection against oxidative stress and work efficiently in the elimination of toxins at the same time. Tulsi is known as Holy Basil or Indian Basil, and is available at international food stores. This recipe makes one serving.

Ingredients:

-8 tulsi leaves

-1 teaspoon of dried green tea leaves

-1 teaspoon of honey

Directions:

1.Wash the tulsi leaves thoroughly before chopping them up.

2.Place the chopped tulsi leaves and dried green tea leaves in a cup.

3.Boil water in a kettle. Let it sit for a few minutes and allow it to cool a bit.

4.Pour the heated water into the cup, cover and let it steep for 3 to 5 minutes.

5.Strain the tea and stir in honey. Enjoy this drink warm or cold.

Green Minty Tea

This tea mixture promotes weight loss by making you feel full, thereby preventing hunger cravings. It also fires up digestion and speeds up fat burning at only 9 calories a cup! This recipe makes one serving.

Ingredients:

-1/2 cup of fresh mint leaves

-1 to 2 teaspoons of dried green tea leaves

-1 teaspoon of honey

Directions:

1.Wash the mint leaves thoroughly before chopping them up.

2.Put the chopped mint and dried green tea leaves in a glass.

3.Boil water in a kettle. Let it sit for a few minutes and allow it to cool a bit.

4.Pour the heated water into the cup, cover and let it steep for 3 to 5 minutes.

5.Put the glass in the fridge. Keep it refrigerated for about 3 to 4 hours.

6.Strain the tea and stir in honey. Drink up for a flat belly!

Fruit and vegetable Infused Green Tea

This combination tea adds variety to your green tea habit. It makes use of cucumber, strawberries and lemon to ensure proper cleansing. This recipe makes 1 serving.

Ingredients:

-2 cups of water

-1 teaspoon of honey

-2 teaspoons of dried green tea leaves

-2 slices of cucumber

-2 strawberries, sliced

-1 slice of lemon

Directions:

1.Boil 2 cups of water in a kettle over medium high heat. Set aside to cool for 3 minutes.

2.Add dried green tea leaves to the hot water. Allow it to steep for 5 minutes.

3.Strain the tea mixture and pour into a tall glass.

4.Stir in the honey and add the strawberry, lemon and cucumber slices.

5.Keep in the fridge for at least 2 hours before serving.

*Chilling the mixture does not only provide you with a refreshingly cool drink, it also helps ensure that the flavors and nutrients from the ingredients are completely infused.

Rosy Green Tea Petals

Aromatic, tasty and healthy, this tea concoction makes it easier for your body to burn calories. This recipe makes one serving.

Ingredients:

-Dried orange rind

-1 teaspoon of dried green tea leaves

-1 teaspoon of dried and crumbled hibiscus and rose petals

Directions:

1.With a vegetable peeler, scrape the rind from the orange. Set it aside to dry at room temperature for an entire day. Once dried, grind the orange rind until fine.

2.Put the ground orange rind, flower petals and dried green tea leaves in a glass.

3.Boil water in a kettle. Let it sit for a few minutes and allow it to cool a bit.

4.Pour the heated water into the cup, cover and let it steep for 10 minutes.

5.Strain the mixture and put it in the fridge to chill for an hour.

6.Stir in honey and enjoy!

Cranberry Tea Spritzer

This is another refreshing drink that will not only quench your thirst but also help you manage your weight more effectively. This concoction makes 4 servings.

Ingredients:

-1/3 cup of water

-3 cups of chilled seltzer

-1/2 cup of cranberry juice

-2 teaspoons of dried green tea leaves

Directions:

1.Boil water in a kettle. Let it sit for a few minutes and allow it to cool a bit.

2.Pour the heated water into the cup over the dried green tea leaves. Let it steep for 3 to 5 minutes.

3.Strain the mixture and let it cool.

4.Pour the tea mixture along with the cranberry juice into a glass pitcher. Stir it well.

5.Pour in a glass and top with the chilled seltzer. Enjoy!

Green Tea Smoothie

A twist to your typical green tea drink, this smoothie combines the nutritious goodness of blueberries, tea, flax seeds and almonds. All of which are known for their weight loss benefits. This yummy drink can help you get rid of belly fat by speeding up metabolism and boosting fat burning abilities.

Ingredients:

-3/4 cup of water

-3 ice cubes

-2 tablespoons of flax seeds

-2 tablespoons of dry roasted almonds, unsalted

-12 ounces of plain yogurt, fat free variety

-2 cups of frozen blueberries

-1 to 2 teaspoons of dried green tea leaves

Directions:

1.Boil water in a kettle. Let it sit for a few minutes and allow it to cool a bit.

2.Pour the heated water into the cup over the dried green tea leaves. Let it steep for 3 to 5 minutes.

3.Strain the mixture and put it in the fridge to chill overnight.

4.Pour all the ingredients along with the green tea mixture in a blender. Process them until smooth. Drink up for a slimmer you!

Fruity Green Smoothie

This combination of fruits, spinach and green tea is a surefire way of burning fat and keeping them away for good! This amazing weight loss recipe drink makes 4 servings.

Ingredients:

-2 cups of ice cubes

-1/2 cup of packed baby spinach

-3 ripe kiwifruits, peeled and cut into 4 equal pieces

-1/2 teaspoon of grated lime rind

-1/4 cup of honey

-3/4 cup of plain yogurt, fat free variety

-2 1/2 cups of frozen diced mangoes

Directions:

1. Boil water in a kettle. Let it sit for a few minutes and allow it to cool a bit.

2. Pour the heated water into the cup over the dried green tea leaves. Let it steep for 3 to 5 minutes.

3. Strain the mixture and set aside to cool.

4. Pour mango, 2 tablespoons of honey, lime rind, 2 tablespoons of water and 1/2 cup of yogurt in a blender. Process until smooth.

5. Fill 4 tall glasses with this first mixture, half full.

6. Wash the blender. Toss in the remaining ingredients along with the tea mixture. Blend the mixture thoroughly.

7. Top off the mango mixture with this tea mixture. Garnish with kiwi slices and enjoy pure goodness!

Conclusion

Thank you again for downloading this book!

I hope this book was able to help you to understand how to detox with tea to derive a wide array of benefits.

The next step is to implement what you have learnt.

If you particularly liked reading about Matcha green tea and would like to either find out more or experience its benefits for yourself, then make sure you visit – www.rawbear.co.uk.

Thank you and good luck!

www.ingramcontent.com/pod-product-compliance
Lightning Source LLC
Chambersburg PA
CBHW062135020426
42335CB00013B/1227